FITNESS PROGRAM

with
SPI

D1280438

PAUL C. BI .D., Ph.D.
LIFE EXTENSION SPECIALIST
and
PATRICIA BRAGG, Ph.D.
Health & Fitness Expert

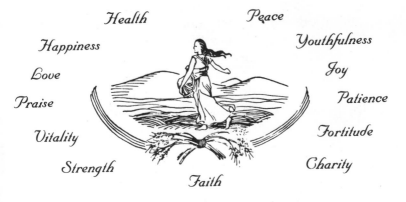

Health   *Peace*

Happiness   *Youthfulness*

Love   *Joy*

Praise   *Patience*

Vitality   *Fortitude*

Strength   *Charity*

Faith

<u>JOIN</u>

The Bragg Crusades for a 100% Healthy, Vigorous, Strong America and a Better World for All!

HEALTH SCIENCE
Box 7, Santa Barbara, California 93102 U.S.A.

FITNESS PROGRAM

with
SPINE MOTION

By
PAUL C. BRAGG, N.D., Ph.D.
LIFE EXTENSION SPECIALIST
and
PATRICIA BRAGG, N.D., Ph.D.
LIFE EXTENSION NUTRITIONIST

- REVISED -
Copyright © Health Science

Thirteenth printing MCMXCII
ISBN: 0-87790-054-X

Published in the United States by
HEALTH SCIENCE - Box 7, Santa Barbara, Calif. 93102, USA

FOREWORD

A PERFECTLY-ALIGNED, FLEXIBLE SPINE
IS IMPORTANT FOR AN ACTIVE, HEALTHY LIFE!

A perfectly-aligned, fully flexible spine is one of the best "head-starts" on perfect health almost all can enjoy! Although we might think that we are born into this world with a perfect spine, it isn't always true!

Unfortunately, even as early as the moment of birth itself, the process of damage to the spine is begun. Authorities say that many physicians grab the baby's head as it emerges during birth, twisting the head up and down to bring out the baby's shoulders, stressing and twisting the tiny spine. During this process a number of spinal misalignments and/or slight breaks can happen, interfering with the child's health thereafter and possibly contributing to sudden infant crib death. Also, if the baby is hung by its feet and slapped on the bottom, a whiplash injury at the base of the skull may occur, causing even more damage...*Read up on the alternate, gentler, more natural birth methods that are available in your area.*

Further misalignments (known as subluxations) happen during childhood years through spankings, falls, fistfights, and the typical wrenching and twisting of limbs encountered by a normal active child. Sports injuries during the teenage years take their toll on the young spine. As adults, poor eating, sleeping, and poor posture habits reinforce all that has gone before, culminating not only in a painful back, but also preventing enjoyment of perfect health! The vital nerves leading from the spinal cord to all other organs in the body haven't ever had a chance to function at their healthy best, because vertebrae of the spinal column have been pressing on them and interfering with their important function. Many times, a general tendency to disease or weak spots in an overall healthy constitution can be traced to such spinal misalignments.

With the simple, gentle Bragg Spine Motion Exercises, many of the effects of a lifetime of inattention and neglect of the spine can be reversed dramatically within a few months, weeks, or even a few days!

Your family Chiropractor can easily diagnose and correct any serious spinal misalignments that, without your suspecting it, may be adversely affecting your overall health and hindering your natural defenses against disease!

Practicing the easy Bragg Fitness Program with Spine Motion is one of the best "preventive maintenance" efforts you can make for your health. These simple exercises and health program will indeed help you live longer, live stronger . . . with a flexible, more painfree back for life.

Live with enthusiasm and your days and life will be filled with more joy, health and happiness! – Patricia Bragg

HEALING HEALTH THERAPIES AND
MASSAGE TECHNIQUES

Explore a few of these wonderful natural methods of healing the body; then choose the technique that's best for your health needs.

F. Mathius Alexander Technique — Lessons intended to end improper use of neuromuscular system and bring body posture back into balance. Eliminates psycho-physical interferences, helps release long-held tension, and aids in re-establishing muscle tone.

Chiropractic — Daniel David Palmer founded chiropractic in 1885 in Davenport, Iowa. From 16 schools now in the U.S., graduates are joining Health Practitioners in all the civilized nations of the world to share their health-healing techniques. Chiropractic is the largest of the non-drug healing professions. Treatment involves soft tissue adjustment and accupressure to free the nervous system of interferences with normal body function. Its concern is the functional integrity of the muscular skeletal system. In addition to manual methods, chiropractors use physical therapy modalities, exercise, health and nutritional guidance.

Feldenkrais Method — Founded by Dr. Moshe Feldenkrais in late 1940s. Lessons lead to improved posture and help create ease and efficiency of movement. A great stress removal method.

Homeopathy — Developed by Dr. Samuel Hahnemann in the 1800s, patients are treated with minute amounts of substances similar to those that cause a particular disease to trigger the body's own defenses. The homeopathic principle is "Like cures like." It is becoming more popular worldwide because it's inexpensive and has minimal side effects.

Naturopathy — Brought to America by Dr. Benedict Lust, M.D., treatment utilizes herbs, diet, fasting, exercise, hydrotherapy, manipulation and sunlight. (Dr. Paul Bragg was a graduate of Dr. Lust's first Naturopathic School in the U.S.) Practitioners reject surgery and drugs except as a last resort.

Osteopathy — The first School of Osteopathy was founded in 1892 by Dr. Andrew Taylor Still, M.D. There are now 15 such colleges in the United States. Treatment involves soft tissue adjustments that free the nervous system from interferences which can cause illness. The complete system of healing by adjustment also includes good nutrition, physical therapies, proper breathing and good posture. Dr. Still's premise was that structure and function of the human body are interdependent and if the structure of the body is altered or abnormal, function is altered and illness results.

(Continued on page 41)

D

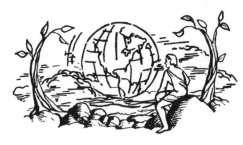

CONTENTS

To maintain good health the body must be exercised properly (walking, jogging, running, biking, swimming, deep breathing, good posture, etc.) and nourished wisely (natural foods), so as to provide and increase the good life of radiant health, joy and happiness. — Paul C. Bragg

CONTENTS

◊◊

It's never too late to begin getting into shape, but it does take daily, sometimes painful perseverance.
—Thomas K. Cureton, Educator

Good health, generated by physical fitness, is the logical starting point for the pursuit of excellence in any field. Physical vitality promotes mental vitality and thus is essential to executive achievement.
—Dr. Richard E. Dutton, Univ. of So. Florida

The True Fountain of Youth - *to look 35 when 60 is ample exercise and healthy foods - these are the tools to prevent heart problems! They also help maintain denser, healthier bone structure.* — Paul C. Bragg

THE FITNESS PROGRAM WITH SPINE MOTION

"Oh, my aching back!"

This cry has echoed down the corridors of time for countless centuries, ever since man learned to stand on his own two feet. This unique accomplishment . . . achieved, among all the varied forms of life on Earth, only by the human species . . . has given mankind the mobility and dexterity to cope with every type of environment found on this planet. It has enabled him to dominate other creatures . . . to "conquer the Earth" . . . and now to set out on the exploration of outer space to conquer other worlds.

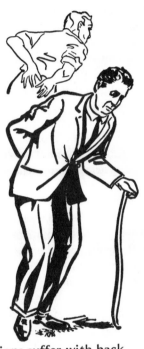

But, as with everything in Nature, there is a price to pay. While scientists debate whether *homo erectus* made his advent hundreds of thousands or millions of years ago, this unique product of creative evolution is still learning how to stand erect! From babyhood on, every human being repeats the evolutionary process . . . wiggler, crawler, toddler, walker, runner . . . and all through life must pay attention to his posture . . . or suffer from backache and its related ills.

Millions suffer with back pains needlessly! Start your Spine Motion Program Today.

THE SPINE AS A KEY TO HEALTH

Universal native folklore equates "backbone" with courage . . . an intuitive tribute to erect posture and the key role of the spine in physical fitness. Physical fitness is more than muscular power. It is the superior condition of the human body. When your body is fit and every muscle and organ is functioning properly, that body becomes a power-house of vim and vigor. Physical fitness means more than just plain health. It means more than the absence of illness ... it means no hidden liabilities, no silent, painless illness working away like termites in the organic framework of the human house. And the "ridgepole" of the human house is the spine.

Let us summarize briefly the key role of the spine in almost every function of the human body. It is the pivot of the skeleton, the framework of bones which gives the body its shape. Anchored to the spine are layers of large and small muscles and ligaments of the back and abdomen, essential in holding the body erect and the vital organs in place ... and these organs themselves are supported by the spine. In four-footed and four-handed creatures, the vital organs are suspended downward from a curved spinal column ... but in two-footed, two-handed man they must be held up against the pull of gravity by an erect spinal column.

And in the center of that column, descending directly from the base of the brain and protected by the bony vertebrae, is the spinal cord ... the "control center" of extensive, intricate networks of motor and sensory nerves that radiate to all parts of the body.

For these basic reasons, which will be discussed in detail during the course of this book, I believe that many ills can be traced to an abnormal spine. For example, prolonged habits of incorrect posture ... as well as sudden movement, jolt or strain ... can cause a vertebra to shift slightly out of alignment (become subluxated) and to press against a nerve passing out from the spinal cord through an opening at that level. Such an impingement is an open invitation to trouble in the organ or part of the body serviced by that partially pinched nerve.

For similar reasons the spine itself is often thrown out of alignment ... into abnormal curves toward the sides, front or back ... which adversely affect other bones of the skeleton, shorten or stretch muscles and ligaments, cause organs to prolapse (fall), and bring on interrelated malfunctions throughout the body.

ORIGINATOR OF SPINE MOTION EXERCISES

To help alleviate such conditions as mentioned above and others arising from structural defects of the spine, and thus to help the body restore itself to natural health, I originated the Spine Motion Exercises which I will give you in this book.

At the time these were introduced some 60 or more years ago, press and public reception was so enthusiastic, that claims made by those

2

who used these exercises sounded extravagant. Only a small part of the amazing results reported would have to be true to establish the principle of Spine Motion as the valuable force it is.

As remarkable as may be the results attained by you and others in following these Spine Motion Exercises, I do not want anyone to regard this as evidence that these exercises can supplant all other health measures. They cannot, and they are not intended to. You must follow a well rounded health program, including proper nutrition, adequate rest, and other forms of exercise . . . all of which will also be discussed in this book.

Nor are Spine Motion Exercises to be considered as a "cure" for any condition, illness or disease. In fact, Nature has no "cures" in the generally accepted sense of the word. The human body is self-healing and self-repairing when we work with Nature, not against her. If we feel sick and miserable, we have brought this condition upon ourselves by our failure to obey natural laws.

The Bragg Spine Motion Exercises are a natural, drugless approach to natural health. They are designed to help restore the spine to its natural, normal functions . . . and thereby help eliminate the causes of many apparent ailments in the back and other parts of the body which arise primarily from defects in the spinal structure . . . defects brought on by habitually poor posture, flabby muscles, improper living and working habits, accidents and injuries.

If you are now under medical care, by all means consult your doctor about the special exercises and general health program presented in this book. Many orthopedists, neurologists, family physicians, osteopaths, as well as physiotherapists and chiropractors, have found it helpful to their patients.

REMARKABLE RESULTS WITH SPINE MOTION

I have seen back injuries and displacements, resulting from a fall, slip, coughing, sneezing or other sudden movement, respond wonderfully to these Spine Motion Exercises. Occupational accidents . . . such as sprains and strains from improper lifting, pulling, carrying or bending . . . often produce the type of pain and misery that only Spine Motion Exercises can relieve.

At one time when I returned from a lecture tour I found my brother in great pain. He had been preparing a piece of ground to plant an organic vegetable garden and came across a large, heavy stone. Not

3

realizing how very heavy it was, he strained or sprained his back in trying to lift it.

Unable to continue his work because of severe, crippling back pain, he had been taking all kinds of treatments ... but the condition persisted. I advised him to take a very hot bath each day, and immediately after the bath to start very lightly doing my Spine Motion Exercises.

He followed my advice, doing the very simple exercises at first ... gradually progressing to the more strenuous ones. At the end of one week his pains were gone ... and in another week he was once more working in his organic garden.

I have known cases of severe injuries to the back, such as whiplash in auto accidents, in which great relief was attained by lightly performing simple Spine Motion Exercises. And I have helped many an athlete back to normal after a severe back injury, especially in such physically punishing sports as basketball, wrestling and ice hockey.

A lifelong athlete myself, I have engaged in all types of sports. I believe that it has been my daily practice of the Spine Motion Exercises which has so strengthened my spine that I have never had serious back injuries, even though I have had some bad spills.

I receive letters from people all over the world who have followed the instructions given in this book, and have found relief from pain in such conditions as lumbago, sacroiliac pain and postural defects of long duration ... as well as painful cases of bursitis (inflammation of the bursa, especially of the shoulder, elbow and knee joints), sciatica, arthritis, and persistent headaches.

MOST PEOPLE'S SPINES ARE DEFECTIVE

About 1 of every 150 persons of average development has a sufficiently flexible spine. In our present society the vast majority of people are sedentary, warping their spines by faulty posture habits in sitting, standing and walking and by general lack of exercise, as well as improper diet. This applies not only to adults, but also to school children of the "TV generation" and modern schools that do not require basic "physical ed."

A recent study of teenagers in the 7th and 8th grades reports 11% with scoliosis, or spinal curvature. The research was conducted among 841 students in Downey, California, by Dr. Leon Brooks, an orthopedic surgeon in the spine deformities service of Rancho Los Amigos Hospital, who expects to continue this study to include some 20,000 adolescents. Dr. Brooks noted that untreated scoliosis can be responsible in later life for back pains and respiratory problems. Special exercises are the basic treatment, except in severe cases which may require braces or even surgery.

Sporadic and incorrect exercise also takes toll of the spine . . . as well as overly strenuous exercise, as among construction workers and athletes.

From the thousands of cases on record in my files, let me cite three illustrative examples:

One is the case of a boy whose spine was so badly slumped that it disturbed his nervous reflexes to the point that he could not take part in the ordinary play and games of youth. After four weeks of Bragg Spine Motion Exercises, he became normally active . . . and later developed into a remarkable swimmer.

Another is a logger of the north woods, who at age 55 was forced to abandon his rigorous outdoor work because of subluxation of the spine (partial dislocation of some of the vertebrae). He was puttering at odd jobs around the camp, when he started the Spine Motion Exercises. In less than a month, he was able to resume logging. Here was a man who for years had swung an axe, surely a vigorous form of exercise! Even so, the spine had become defective because of lack of extension in the right directions and to the right degree. It required the peculiar, anatomical twist of the more scientific Spine Motion to align and flex his spine at every point.

A third case is that of a 43-year-old woman who was apparently headed for invalidism, with organs supposedly far out of place and ailments which had baffled ordinary forms of correction. After a few days of practicing the Spine Motion Exercises, she obtained complete relief.

SPINE MOTION SIMPLE AND SCIENTIFIC

The three cases just described are widely diverse . . . yet all three responded beneficially to the same Spine Motion Exercises. Why?

Remember that the spinal column is the focus of the skeletal, muscular and nervous systems. Even a slight dislocation or malfunction in the spine can affect other parts of the body.

A scientific study of the spinal structure has made it possible to devise simple motions which give the spine the requisite "pull" or

5

stretch to restore its natural alignment and flexibility. The effects of such motions have been carefully recorded and compared. It has been found that these simple manipulations . . . through careful, active use of the trunk muscles . . . cause all the tiny bones comprising the spinal column to separate normally and allow Nature to build up the cushiony growths of cartilage between each pair of bones.

Life holds many everyday examples of what resilience means to any mechanism. Imagine an automobile without springs, a piano without felt hammers, a typewriter without the yielding rubber platen and soft, resilient feet to dispel vibration.

In thinking of anything mechanical, just recall that every machine ever designed is patterned after the master mechanism constituting the human body. The more perfect the machine, the closer its designers have come to the principles of motion found in the human body.

Dr. Morris Fishbein, late and long-time head of the American Medical Association, stated:

"Fortunately for mankind, the back has developed so well that it is capable of withstanding stresses and strains better than many other parts of the body. There are some who insist that the back is the weakest part of man. Actually, it is one of the strongest and best. If it could be given the same amount of personal consideration and attention that we give regularly to the teeth, the skin, and other portions of the body that are more easily visible, the human body would be a more efficient working mechanism and one that would last much longer without breaking down."

Let us examine the "mainspring" of this human mechanism, the spine . . . its structure and functions . . . and find out how we can give it the care and attention it needs to fulfill its built-in potential of at least 100 years of good service.

THE SPINE AND THE SKELETAL SYSTEM

If you suddenly removed the poles from a circus tent, the tent would collapse. The spine and the other bones of the human skeleton support the softer parts of the body and give the body its general shape. If the spine, corresponding to the main pole of the tent, and the other supporting bones or "poles" were suddenly removed, the body would sink to the ground in a shapeless mass.

Although a human being may be born with as many as 350 bones,

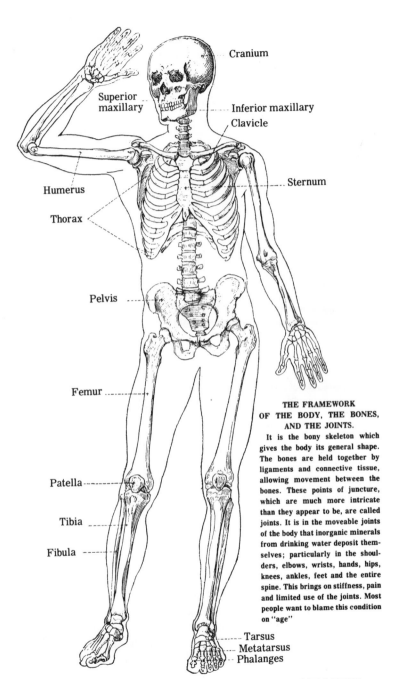

Cranium

Superior maxillary

Inferior maxillary

Clavicle

Sternum

Humerus

Thorax

Pelvis

Femur

Patella

Tibia

Fibula

THE FRAMEWORK OF THE BODY, THE BONES, AND THE JOINTS.

It is the bony skeleton which gives the body its general shape. The bones are held together by ligaments and connective tissue, allowing movement between the bones. These points of juncture, which are much more intricate than they appear to be, are called joints. It is in the moveable joints of the body that inorganic minerals from drinking water deposit themselves; particularly in the shoulders, elbows, wrists, hands, hips, knees, ankles, feet and the entire spine. This brings on stiffness, pain and limited use of the joints. Most people want to blame this condition on "age"

Tarsus
Metatarsus
Phalanges

THE BONES OF THE HUMAN BODY. FRONT VIEW.

7

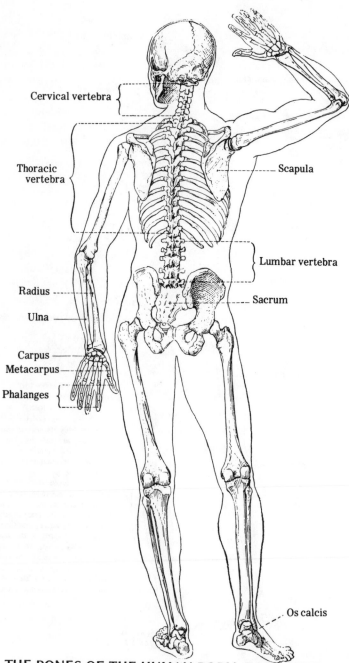

Cervical vertebra

Thoracic
vertebra

Scapula

Lumbar vertebra

Radius

Sacrum

Ulna

Carpus

Metacarpus

Phalanges

Os calcis

THE BONES OF THE HUMAN BODY. BACK VIEW.

many of these grow together as the child develops. A normal adult skeletal system is composed of 206 bones.

The spinal column, the master bones of the human body, is composed of 26 hollow cylinders of bone called vertebrae. If you strung together 26 spools of thread on a stiff wire in the shape of a very open Letter S, you would have constructed something that looks much like the human spinal column. We will discuss its structure in detail later.

The skull, which is supported by the spinal column, is made up of 29 flat bones. The round part of the skull, which encases the brain, is called the cranium and consists of 8 bones. The face, including the lower jaw, consists of 14 bones. There are 3 tiny bones in each ear. In the throat there is a single bone, the hyoid.

The chest is composed of 25 bones . . . a single breast bone, called the sternum . . . and 24 ribs, all of which are attached to the spinal column. The upper 7 pairs of ribs (14 bones) are attached to the spinal column at the back and the sternum in front. The next 3 pairs (6 bones) attach only to the spinal column, curve around the front of the thorax (chest) but do not meet the sternum. The 2 lowest pairs of ribs (4 bones), called the floating ribs, extend from the spine only part way toward the front.

There are two collar bones, or clavicles, which are attached to the sternum in front and to the two shoulder blades (scapula) at each side.

Each arm consists of one upper arm bone, the humerus, and two forearm bones, the ulna and the radius. There are 8 bones in each wrist, the carpals, each with a different anatomical name and function. Five bones, called metacarpals, connect the wrist with the fingers, which are composed of 14 bones, called phalanges (2 in the thumb, 3 in each of the other four fingers).

Connected to the lowest part of the spinal column, the sacrum and coccyx, are the two hip bones (coxa), the broadest bones of the skeleton. Each connects with a thigh bone (femur), the thigh bones being the longest, strongest and heaviest bones of the body. In each leg the kneecap (patella) covers the joint attaching the thigh bone to the two lower leg bones, the shinbone (tibia) and its smaller companion, the fibula.

There are 7 bones in each ankle, the tarsals, larger than those in the wrist. Five bones, called metatarsals, form the arch of the foot, connecting the ankle and toes. As in the fingers, there are 14 bones (also called phalanges) in the toes of each foot, 2 in the great toe and 3 in each of the others.

JOINTS AND CARTILAGE

Except for the U-shaped hyoid bone of the throat, every bone in the body is connected, or articulates, with another . . . the spinal column being the pivot of the entire skeletal system.

The point at which two bones meet, or articulate, is known as a joint. The joints of the cranium, that part of the skull which houses the brain, are immovable. Those joining the ribs and the spine are partially movable. Movement is even more limited in the sacroiliac joints, connecting the base of the spine with the hip bones, where the whole weight of the trunk is supported. Sacroiliac pain occurs when the tough, resistant ligaments, which hold these joints firmly in place, weaken under continued or unusual stress . . . such as lifting heavy objects or a sudden twisting of the body or straining to raise a window that is jammed. (Spine Motion Exercises help to strengthen these important ligaments.)

There are four main types of movable joints in the body . . . and, as you will recognize from their names, these human joints have served as patterns which man has adapted mechanically. Permitting the widest

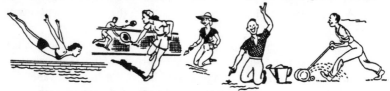

KEEP YOUNG BIOLOGICALLY
WITH EXERCISE AND GOOD NUTRITION

You can always remember that you have the following good reasons for sticking to your health program:

- The ironclad laws of Nature.
- Your common sense which tells you that you are doing right.
- Your aim to make your health better and your life longer.
- Your resolve to prevent illness so that you may enjoy life.
- By making an art of life, you will be young at any age.
- You will retain your faculties and be hale, hearty, active and useful far beyond the ordinary length of days, and you will also possess superior mental and physical powers.

Healthy Exercise Habit: As I stride along on my daily two mile brisk walk, I say to myself – often out loud – "Health, Strength, Youth, Vitality, Understanding, Peace, Love, Joy and Salvation for Eternity." It amazes me daily how our wonderful Lord fills my life with all His glorious blessings!
– Patricia Bragg

range of movement are those connecting the shoulders and upper arm bones, and the hips and thigh bones, known as ball-and-socket joints. Hinge joints, such as those of the knees, fingers and toes, allow bending back and forth only. A pivot joint permits the bones to rotate at the joint like a key turning in a lock, such as at wrists and ankles and the joints at the base of fingers and toes. The elbow is a combination of pivot joint and hinge joint, allowing one bone of the forearm to rotate about the other as well as a bending motion.

The vertebral joints of the spinal column are known as saddle joints, permitting limited movement forward, backward and sidewise. Although each vertebra moves only slightly on the one adjoining it, the combined movements of the 26 bones make the whole column flexible.

Nature provides lubrication for these movable joints with a substance called synovial fluid, permanently encased in a membrane. The natural supply of this fluid is ample for a lifetime, but proper diet is important in maintaining its consistency ... particularly the avoidance

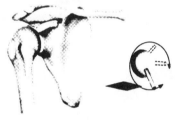
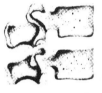
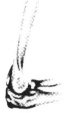

Ball-and-socket joints at hips and shoulders permit freest movement of all body joints. Hips and shoulders are examples.

The vertebrae are saddle joints, moving forward, backward, and sidewise. One vertebra moves only slightly on the next, but the whole column is fairly flexible.

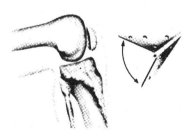
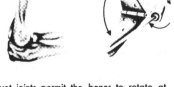

Hinge joints are like the hinges you know—permitting backward and forward movement only, like the hinges of a door. Your knees and your fingers are hinge joints.

Pivot joints permit the bones to rotate at the joint like a key turning in a lock. The elbow is a combination of pivot joint and hinge joint. Thanks to this joint one bone of the forearm can rotate about the other.

of hard drinking water and other substances containing inorganic minerals, as will be discussed in a later section of this book.

Also lining the bone surfaces of the joints is a tough, springy tissue called cartilage ... which not only prevents the bone surfaces from rubbing against each other, but also acts as an all-important shock absorber. This is particularly important in the spine, where cartilage

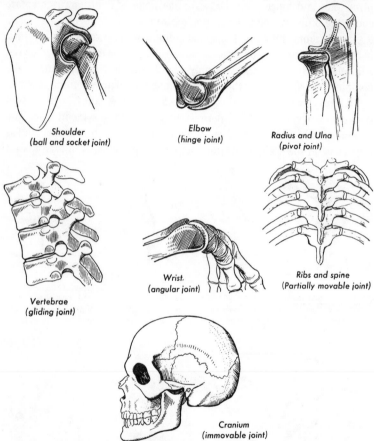

Shoulder
(ball and socket joint)

Elbow
(hinge joint)

Radius and Ulna
(pivot joint)

Vertebrae
(gliding joint)

Wrist.
(angular joint)

Ribs and spine
(Partially movable joint)

Cranium
(immovable joint)

These are the types of joints in your body that have movement. Between each of these moveable joints there is a clear amber fluid called synovial fluid which acts as a lubricant to keep the joints moving easily. When inorganic minerals from drinking water and toxic acid crystals replace this synovial fluid we have stiffness, pain and misery.

plates and intervertabral disks (described later) between the vertebrae absorb the shocks of ordinary actions such as walking and sitting, as well as blows to the spine.

Cartilage is the precursor of bones in the formation of the skeleton in the embryo, and some of it remains as part of the skeletal system. At birth, the "soft" parts of a baby's skull are cartilaginous, to allow room for growth of the brain, changing into hard bone like the rest of the skull after the brain has attained full size. Since cartilage is more elastic than rigid bone, some of it remains at the juncture of the ribs and the sternum to allow full lung expansion. Cartilage also remains part of the adult skeleton in semi-rigid tubes which must be kept permanently open . . . such as the larynx, trachea (windpipe), bronchi, nose and ears.

Cartilage, which is also called "gristle," is often confused with tendons and ligaments. All three are tough, white tissues with varying degrees of elasticity and differences in structure and functions. Cartilage is "embryonic bone" but has no direct blood supply . . . it is semi-rigid but elastic. Tendons are the white, glistening fibrous bands which attach muscles to bones . . . with great tensile strength but non-elastic . . . containing a few blood vessels and sensory nerves. Ligaments are of similar structure but contain elastic fibers . . . connect two or more bones or cartilages . . . support certain organs, muscles and fascia (fibrous enveloping tissue).

Tendons and ligaments are part of the muscular system . . . while cartilage is part of the skeletal system.

COMPOSITION OF THE BONES

To be healthy and strong, both cartilage and bones need a full daily ration of organic calcium, phosphorus, magnesium and manganese . . . and natural sources of these important minerals will be given in a later section on Nutrition.

The long bones, such as those of the arms and legs, are generally cylindrical in shape. The long cylindrical portion is called the shaft. The ends of these bones are thicker than the shaft, and are shaped to fit into the ends of the adjoining bones to form the various types of joints described in the preceding section. The short bones, such as those of the wrist and ankle, are composed mostly of a thick shaft of elastic, spongy material inside a thin covering of hard bone material. Flat bones, such as the ribs, are made up of spongy material between plates of hard bone.

A cross section of bone shows the two main types of material of which it is composed. The hard outer material, which gives the bone its shape and strength, consists primarily of chemical compounds of calcium and phosphorous. The bones and teeth contain 90% of the body's calcium, which is required for repair of body tissues more than any other mineral.

The soft inner part of the bone is called marrow. Most bone marrow is yellowish in color . . . made up of fat cells, and serving as a storage depot for fat which can be converted into energy as the body's needs require. Toward the ends of the long bones and generally throughout the interior of the flat bones, such as those of the skull and the spinal column, patches and streaks of reddish tissue show in the marrow. These are the vital manufacturing centers of the red blood cells, or corpuscles, which transport life-giving oxygen throughout the body. The white blood corpuseles, which combat infection, are also produced in the bone marrow.

PROTECTION OF THE VITAL ORGANS

The bones also help to protect the softer parts of the body, especially the vital organs. The skull forms a strong case for the soft gray matter of the brain. Two bony sockets in front of the skull protect the eyes. The spinal column forms a bony tube that safeguards the delicate, vital spinal cord.

The ribs form a hard, elastic framework that protects the heart and lungs. If a person had no ribs and bumped into something, even a small bump might collapse the lungs or damage the heart. The lower rib cage also shelters, at back and sides, the kidneys and major organs of the upper digestive system. As noted, the ribs are supported by the spinal column.

The pelvic bones, which include the base of the spinal column (sacrum and coccyx) and the hip bones, provide protection for the bladder and the reproductive organs.

STRUCTURE OF THE SPINAL COLUMN

How is this marvelous pivot of the human skeleton constructed? Although, to illustrate some of its functions, we have likened it to the ridgepole of a house or the main pole of a tent, the spine is not a single rigid bone . . . if it were, the motions of the human body would be very limited.

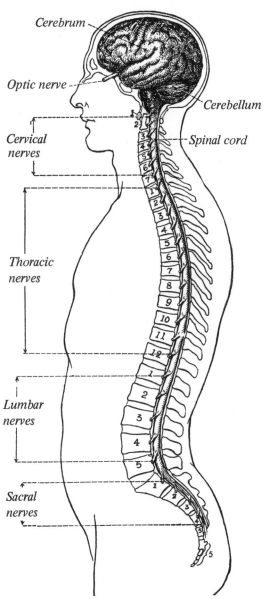

Cerebrum

Optic nerve

Cervical
nerves

Cerebellum

Spinal cord

Thoracic
nerves

Lumbar
nerves

Sacral
nerves

GENERAL VIEW OF THE CENTRAL NERVOUS SYSTEM AND SPINE
It is in the cushions between the bones of the spine that the inorganic minerals
from water may deposit themselves and cause back aches, slipped discs and
many other problems of the spine. Nerve force to the vital organs may be greatly
lessened, bringing on many painful miseries throughout the entire body.

The spine is a flexible column composed of 26 bones . . . 24 small vertebrae from the base of the skull to the pelvic region . . . the sacrum, which is actually the natural fusion of 5 embryonic vertebrae into a wedge-shaped bone that forms the back of the pelvis . . . and the coccyx, or "tail bone," a small triangular bone of 4 fused embryonic vertebrae at the base of the sacrum. (NOTE: During its growth inside the womb, the human embryo first develops 33 vertebrae, the lower 9 fusing into the sacrum and coccyx before birth.)

At birth, the human spine forms a single, arched curve. As the baby begins to lift his head and sit erect, the 7 upper vertebrae between the base of the skull and the shoulders, forming the neck, strengthen into what is known as the cervical curve.

The next 12 vertebrae, to which the ribs are attached at the back of the chest, continue to curve outward. These are known as the thoracic vertebrae (chest = thorax), and are larger than the cervical because they have a heavier load to support.

When the baby begins to stand erect and to walk, the next 5 vertebrae adjust to form the inward lumbar curve, the "small of the back." The sacrum curves backward again, attaching at the sacroiliac joints to the hip bones . . . and the little coccyx completes the spine with an inward turn.

These natural shallow "S" curves of the spinal column are the basis of the resilient strength which makes it the mainspring of the human body. The components of this spring are the vertebrae.

Each vertebra is intricately constructed, with two main parts . . . the body and the spinal arch.

The round body of the vertebra projects inward . . . a solid piece of spongy textured bone which forms the weight bearing part of the spinal column. The top and bottom of each vertebral body is covered with a thin circular plate of cartilage. Between the bodies of each two vertebrae is a cushioning intervertebral disk, a marvelous little mechanism composed of a thin, elastic outside covering of fibrocartilage with a semi-fluid center. These disks, which we shall discuss in more detail later, make it possible for the spinal column to move comfortably in various directions from bending to stretching, and to absorb shocks. If it were not for these disks, you would feel a blow at the base of your skull every time you sat down or took a step.

The spinal arches of the vertebrae form the opening, or canal, for the passage and protection of the spinal cord. At the back of each arch are five fingerlike bony projections, to which the intricate system of back

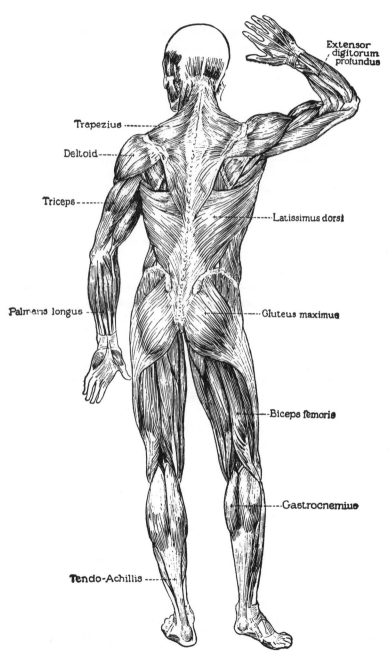

Extensor
digitorum
profundus

Trapezius ------

Deltoid-----

Triceps ------

Palmaris longus -

----------Latissimus dorsi

------- Gluteus maximus

-Biceps femoris

----Gastrocnemius

Tendo-Achillis ----

THE MUSCLES OF THE HUMAN BODY. BACK VIEW.

17

ligaments and muscles are anchored. The central projections, known as spinous processes, are what you feel as your "backbone." Joining the vertebrae are interlocking, gliding joints projecting up and down from each arch and enveloped by capsules lined with synovial fluid.

THE SPINE AND THE MUSCULAR SYSTEM

Although the intervertebral joints add to the flexibility of the spine and help to keep it in alignment, what really holds the spinal column together and in shape are the strong, tough ligaments which weave in and out of the fingerlike projections of the spinal arches. Extending from the skull to the sacrum, these powerful, elastic ligaments lash together all the vertebrae and intervertebral disks. Another system of extremely tough ligaments is woven back and forth throughout the sacroiliac area to give the tremendous support necessary to hold together these joints between the hips and the base of the spine, which must bear most of the human body's weight.

An elaborate system of muscles is also attached to the vertebrae by tendons to help hold the vertebrae in place when the human body is at rest and to allow them to move when it is in motion. It is these muscles and the interwoven ligaments around the spinal column which the Spine Motion Exercises are especially designed to activate . . . to achieve and maintain the full length and flexibility of the spinal column.

Without muscles to operate the levers, sockets, pivots and gliders of the skeletal system, our skeletons would remain a mere assemblage of static bones . . . and just as it is the pivot of the skeletal system, the spinal column is the key anchor point of the muscular system. Layers of powerful muscles of the back and abdomen manipulate the body's major movements . . . bending forward, backward and sidewise . . . reaching upward . . . lifting, carrying . . . pulling, pushing. Movements of the head and neck are accomplished by muscles anchored to upper cervical vertebrae. Shoulder and upper arm muscles anchor to cervical, thoracic and upper lumbar vertebrae, thigh muscles to the sacrum and coccyx.

The muscles operative in our breathing apparatus are anchored to the spine . . . the diaphragm to lumbar vertebrae, rib muscles to thoracic and cervical vertebrae. Pelvic muscles that support the viscera and are important in elimination are anchored to the lower spine.

WHY THE SPINE "SHRINKS"

Even with the operation of all these muscles, the ordinary daily activities of the average person do not fully exercise the spine. Its built-in capacity is seldom, if ever, used ... especially in our under-exercised, malnourished "affluent" society of today. This is a civilization of sitters and spectator sportsmen ... who are overfed and undernourished by devitalized, artificial foods.

Muscles become flabby from lack of exercise ... tissues depleted from lack of proper nourishment. Unused and misused, the spine "settles" ... stiffens ... and often becomes misshapen. Dependent upon exercise and good circulation in adjacent tissues for their nourishment, cartilage and disks between the vertebrae deteriorate. The unstretched spinal column "shrinks" ... many people in their 60's and 70's becoming as much as 3 to 5 inches shorter in height ... and some of them "bent over by old age."

It is not age, however, which causes the spine to shorten or become bent into abnormal curvature. Deficiency in diet and insufficient or incorrect exercise are so prevalent that many of our children and adolescents scuff along with slumped spines and no energy or vitality. The longer this condition persists, of course, the more pronounced it becomes ... that is why it is attributed to age.

If time were the only factor, however, my spine would be fossilized ... as I am a man with grown great-grandchildren. Yet my spine is just as long, just as flexible, just as strong as it was more than half a century ago. Why? Because I know the vital importance of exercising the spinal column to keep the circulation going into my spinal region and to maintain the muscles and ligaments, which hold the spine in place, in top tone and fitness ... and I know the essential value of eating the foods which contain the important minerals and vitamins to build strong, healthy bones and cartilage.

No spine is any stronger than the food material of which it is made ... and no spine is any stronger than the exercise that it is given ... regardless of your calendar years. And nothing affects your entire health, your energy and vitality, as much as the condition of your spinal column.

The three greatest letters in the English alphabet are N-O-W. There is no time like the present. Begin now!

—Sir Walter Scott

YOU CAN HAVE A YOUTHFUL SPINE AT ANY AGE

Bernarr Macfadden, the father of physical culture with whom I began my own career, often said that a person is as young as his spine. "Any man or woman can take thirty years off the age condition by straightening and stretching the spine," he stated.

It is literally so. It has been done and is being done. You can prevent the process called "aging" . . . or repair its inroads on your health . . . to an amazing extent by Spine Motion Exercises and proper nutrition. There is nothing in physiology which responds in so quick and positive a manner as the spinal column when gently but sufficiently extended to its full elastic capacity.

Consider the fact that most people usually feel their best in the morning upon arising. This is not alone from refreshing sleep but also because the spine has lengthened by its long rest. You have often heard that you are "taller" in the morning. By comparative measurements you may easily verify this. But the longer length brought about by repose is very quickly lost, as the upright position and activities of the day cause the spine once again to "settle" . . . unless you have strengthened the spinal column and its supporting ligaments and muscles by a systematic program of exercise and nutrition such as the one given in this book.

Very few people exercise the spine sufficiently, and the cartilage plates and disks become "squeezed." Subjected as it is to constant friction between the vertebrae, cartilage can wear thin and cause painful complications. The disks are subject to degenerative changes such as calcification. As a result, not only do the bony surfaces of the vertebrae rub against each other, but they also impinge on or "pinch" the nerves emerging from the spinal cord through vertebral openings.

Fortunately, cartilage responds readily to the stimulation of Spine Motion Exercises which are designed to stretch the spinal column, opening the natural spacing between the vertebrae. Cartilage grows from the moment it is given room to develop. It is this quick restoration of cartilage that makes it so astonishingly easy to accomplish apparent wonders with Spine Motion Exercises irrespective of the person's age. In fact, age affects cartilage growth less than almost any form of replacement in the body. It is possible to produce abundant cartilage . . . and to have a biologically young spine regardless of your calendar years.

WHAT IS A "SLIPPED DISK"?

The chief shock absorbers of the spinal column and the "ball bearings" which give it such great flexibility and resilience are the intervertebral disks. These little cushions between the vertebrae are composed of a "stuffing" of extremely elastic tissue, about the consistency of a pudding but very tough, called the nucleus pulposus . . . which is encased in a laminated (layered) covering called the annulus, resembling an onion but exceptionally tough and resilient. It is reinforced at top and bottom by the cartilage plates, which protect the disk from contact with the bone.

When the spine flexes, in whatever direction, the disks are compressed in that direction . . . pushing the nucleus in the opposite direction to fill the extra space there between the vertebrae. In a strong, healthy spine the "ball bearing" function of these disks can withstand a great deal of pressure.

However, if the annulus (covering) becomes weakened . . . or if the disk is subjected to severe compression by a sudden jolt or undue strain . . . the pressure on the nucleus pushes it through the outer covering into the spinal canal. In medical terms this is a ruptured intervertebral disk or herniated nucleus pulposus . . . commonly known as a "slipped disk." When this occurs, and the disk is pushed out into the spinal canal, it blocks this passageway and can produce damaging pressure on the vital spinal cord. At the same time the adjoining vertebrae, robbed of this insulating cushion, press against each other and on the nerves emanating from the spinal cord at that point.

Until this injury became so prevalent during World War II . . . primarily from bouncing in jeeps over rugged terrain . . . the resulting severe pain was most frequently diagnosed as sciatica or other known forms of low-back pain. Once the true cause was discovered, however, remedial surgical techniques were developed. These have now become so perfected, as well as methods of diagnosis, that practically normal spinal function can be restored, although the disk itself cannot be replaced or regenerated.

In addition to avoiding sudden or severe strains . . . the best way to avoid a "slipped disk" is to lengthen and strengthen your spine by correct exercise and nourishment, so that your disks will be strong and healthy, tough and resilient.

NEW PAPAIN ENZYME THERAPY HELPS THOUSANDS

Before you consider drastic surgery for your slipped, herniated-ruptured disk . . . you may want to try a more natural alternative. The treatment receiving praise in many slipped disk cases is Chemo-Papain injections performed by a Neuro or Orthopedic Surgeon. This treatment was pioneered in Canada, where thousands of Americans went to receive it . . . until the U.S. government approved the treatment in 1983.

Chemo-Papain injections are saving thousands from drastic back operations. Use of a simple papain enzyme from the papaya seems to work miracles in many cases by helping to smooth out the ruptured areas. The enzyme helps make the area painfree by dissolving the extruded portion of the disk that has become lifeless due to being squeezed, which cuts off the blood supply. Chemo-Papain does not destroy healthy tissue . . . but dissolves only the sick, extruded, ruptured area!

These injections can be given on an out-patient basis requiring only an 8-hour stay in a hospital clinic. A local anesthetic is used to deaden only the area where the injections are to be given. Afterwards, the complete recovery program is important: proper exercise, sound health diet, and proper rest and maintenance of the entire body!

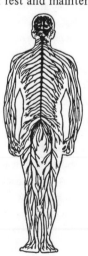

THE NERVOUS SYSTEM IS THE COMMUNICATION SYSTEM OF YOUR BODY

The nervous system is the communication system of your body. It is made up of the brain and nerves which extend throughout the body. Note that the nerves vary considerably in diameter.

THE SPINAL CORD . . . VITAL "CONTROL CENTER"

The most important function of the spine is protection of the spinal cord . . . the vital "control center" without which the skeletal and muscular systems and the vital organs of the body could not operate.

Not even the most sophisticated computer system can match the performance of this cord of nerve tissue. Less than 1-1/2 feet long, little more than 1/3-inch in diameter, and weighing about 1 ounce, the spinal cord is the calculating and relay center of a vast and intricate network of nerves that reach into every part of the human body.

Continuous with and extending downward from the base of the brain, the medulla oblongata, the spinal cord passes through the canal formed by the vertebral arches. At the first lumbar vertebra the single cord ends in a number of delicate filaments or threads which extend to the end of the spine and fasten the cord to the coccyx. Cerebrospinal fluid maintains pressure in the cord, which is insulated from the bony canal by three layers of coverings called meninges.

The spinal nerves pass through openings in the vertebral arches and branch out to serve various parts of the body. There are 31 pairs of these nerves . . . 8 cervical, 12 thoracic, 5 lumbar, 5 sacral and one coccyx. Roots of the sensory nerves, which convey feeling, are attached to the back or dorsal side of the spinal cord . . . and roots of the corresponding motor nerves, controlling action, are attached to the front or ventral side. Each pair controls a specific part of the body. For example, if you stub your toe against a piece of furniture, the branch of the sensory nerve to that leg and foot flashes a pain signal to the central control in the spinal cord . . . and the matching motor nerve immediately transmits the order to pull back your foot. This is done so swiftly that your reaction seems instantaneous.

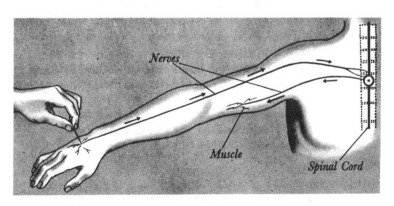

Nerves

Muscle

Spinal Cord

THE PATH THAT A MESSAGE MAY TAKE
IF THE HAND IS PRICKED

Except for those controlled by the 12 cranial (brain) nerves, automatic or reflex actions are controlled by the spinal cord. For example, we "see" in our brain via the cranial optic nerve ... but certain eye muscles are controlled from the spinal cord ... and we "cry" by order of a spinal nerve which controls the lacrimal gland.

Conscious actions originate in the brain ... but when these become reflex, they are usually transferred to the control center of the spinal cord. In computer terminology, the brain "programs" a course of action ... but when it becomes a habit, it becomes part of the "data bank" of the spinal cord. When you learn to drive a car, for example, at first you must consciously think out every move ... but with practice, it becomes automatic. Consider the fact that an experienced driver, when passing another car, automatically calculates the speed of his own car, that of the car to be passed and of any car approaching, and decides how much to accelerate in what length of time in order to pass the car safely. If he had to stop and figure this out consciously, he would never pass the other car! But it is done in a "split second" by his spinal nerve reflexes. The same sort of thing happens in emergencies ... and in countless daily actions, such as walking, eating, talking, etc., which were programmed in infancy. Already in the data bank of our spinal computer at birth was its role in regulating our breathing, heartbeat and circulation, digestion, elimination and reproductive functions.

THE SPINE AND THE NERVOUS SYSTEM

Now you can see why it is so important to keep your spine long, strong and flexible. It is constructed by Nature to protect your vital spinal cord in perfect alignment, with no impingement on it or the spinal nerves ... while also allowing great freedom of body movement in all directions.

It is through our nerves that we experience every physical pleasure or pain. The spine which is kept straight, strong, flexible and elongated allows every set of nerves to function freely.

The spine which has "settled" or shortened has less space between the vertebrae ... crowding the nerves which pass through the openings of the vertebral arches ... and finally causing direct pressure of the bone on the nerve.

When such an impingement occurs in the upper cervical vertebrae, at the base of the head or upper neck, it may bring on headaches. An inch

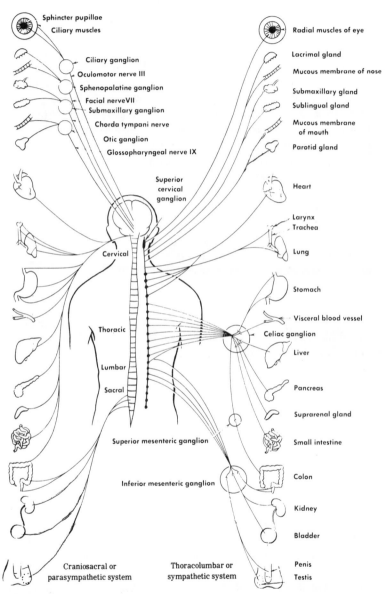

Sphincter pupillae
Ciliary muscles

Radial muscles of eye

Ciliary ganglion
Oculomotor nerve III
Sphenopalatine ganglion
Facial nerve VII
Submaxillary ganglion
Chorda tympani nerve
Otic ganglion
Glossopharyngeal nerve IX

Lacrimal gland
Mucous membrane of nose
Submaxillary gland
Sublingual gland
Mucous membrane of mouth
Parotid gland

Superior cervical ganglion

Heart

Cervical

Larynx
Trachea
Lung

Stomach

Thoracic

Visceral blood vessel
Celiac ganglion
Liver

Lumbar

Sacral

Pancreas

Suprarenal gland

Superior mesenteric ganglion

Small intestine

Inferior mesenteric ganglion

Colon

Kidney

Bladder

Craniosacral or parasympathetic system

Thoracolumbar or sympathetic system

Penis
Testis

The autonomic nervous system showing its two divisions:
the craniosacral or parasympathetic, and the sympathetic.

farther down, and the eye muscles may be strained. In the thoracic area, pressure on nerves to the stomach and/or other digestive organs may cause malfunction or distress there. Farther down, impingement may affect bowels or kidneys. In fact, there is no part of the body, even in the extremity of an arm or leg, which is not affected in some way by the spinal nervous system.

When an accident or injury even slightly displaces a vertebra, the acute pain causes the victim immediately to seek expert treatment.* When the displacement occurs gradually, however, the warning pain is often erroneously attributed to the affected organ or area of the body, rather than to the prime cause of a pinched spinal nerve. The difference is only in degree. A "dislocation" . . . an obvious, violent disarrangement through injury or strain . . . is sudden . . . it is acutely felt. The "settling" process by which a vertebra becomes malpositioned is gradual . . . it may start to grow that way when you are in your teens.

The slow erosion of cartilage and weakening of muscles and ligaments may go unnoticed for a long time, because of the body's amazing natural ability to compensate and the built-in power of the spine to withstand punishment. But when vertebrae have come so close together as to impoverish any set of nerves, some part of the human mechanism slows down, weakens, and draws unduly on nervous vitality in an effort to overcome the handicap.

Nervous energy is so essential to mental and physical health that I would like to recommend, as a companion text to this book, my book on *BUILDING POWERFUL NERVE FORCE.*

Here we are primarily concerned with the spinal column and its relationship to the functioning of that part of the central nervous system controlled by the spinal cord. For peak performance of these nerves, which greatly influence the health of your entire body, a fully flexible, strong, healthy, elongated spine is essential.

----

*

Seek your neighborhood chiropractor who will help you with his specialized knowledge and training in displaced vertebras, back and neck problems. Your chiropractor will help you keep your spine strong, healthy, and in perfect alignment, if you will do your part and keep the muscles strong and healthy by doing these "Spine-Motion" exercises.

We believe in prevention. Your friendly chiropractor is interested in helping you maintain a healthy spine. Therefore it is wise to have your spine checked from time to time by your professional chiropractor.

SPINAL NERVE CENTERS OF
VARIOUS ORGANS OF THE HUMAN BODY

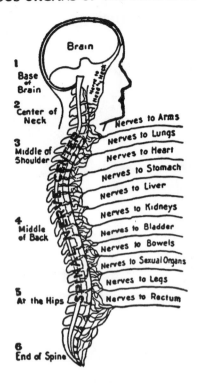

BORON – MIRACLE TRACE MINERAL FOR HEALTHY BONES

BORON – Trace mineral for healthy bones helps the body have more Calcium, Mineral & Hormones! Boron is found in vegetables, fruits, nuts and especially good sources are broccoli, prunes, dates, raisins, almonds, peanuts and soybeans. U.S. Dept. of Agriculture's Human Nutrition Lab in Grand Forks, North Dakota says Boron is always in the soil and in our food, but many Americans eat a low-Boron diet every day. Their recent 17 week study shows with a 3 mg. daily Boron supplement they were able to cut the draining (demineralization) of Calcium, Phosphorus and Magnesium from the body and often caused by the easy, fast food, high meat diet, which most American's suffer from. After only eight weeks on the Boron supplement study Calcium loss was cut by 40%. Boron also helped double certain important Hormones, which are thought to be vital to maintaining Calcium and healthy bone status. Millions of women today are taking estrogen-replacement therapy for Osteoporosis, Boron just might replace this, naturally...along with changing to a 100% healthy lifestyle with ample exercises which helps maintain healthy bones along with a low-fat, high-fiber, high-carbohydrate diet...which science now says may help protect against heart disease, high blood pressure, cancer and more. Happy to see science now agrees with my Dad who stated these simple health truths over 70 years ago.

27

POSTURE SILHOUETTES

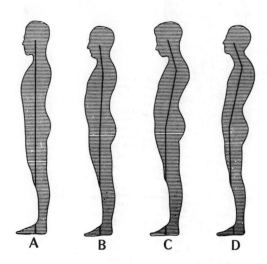

(A) Good: head, trunk, and thigh in straight line; chest high and forward; abdomen flat; back curves normal. (B) Fair: head forward; abdomen prominent; exaggerated curve in upper back; slightly hollow back. (C) Poor: relaxed (fatigue) posture; head forward; abdomen relaxed; shoulder blades prominent; hollow back. (D) Very poor: head forward badly; very exaggerated curve in upper back; abdomen relaxed; chest flat-sloping; hollow back.

PROPER POSTURE . . . THE CONTINUOUS EXERCISE

Before we go into the special Spine Motion Exercises, we must establish the basic exercise which should be so thoroughly programmed into your nervous system that you practice it all the time . . . standing, sitting, walking, lying down. This continuous exercise is the habit of proper posture. It begins in infancy and continues throughout life. As noted previously, the human species is still learning how to maintain an erect posture.

Posture means how we hold our bodies. Proper posture is the balanced alignment of the body. When standing erect, an imaginary plumb line representing the center of gravity should fall in alignment with the top center of the skull through the center of the ear, and through the centers of the joints at the shoulder, hip, knee and ankle. The chin should be right angles to the rest of the body . . . shoulders straight and chest up but not in an exaggerated stance . . . the abdomen firm but not "sucked in." In this position, the spine holds its natural, gentle curves . . . and the weight of the body is supported by the hip joints and the feet, slightly apart, with stress on the heels.

To sum it up, "Stand tall!" To get that tall feeling, imagine that a powerful giant is holding you by the hair and almost lifting you off the ground. You should not only stand tall, but also sit tall and walk tall.

If you have been slouching or slumping, as most people do, you will probably find the erect posture uncomfortable at first, because your muscles and ligaments have become too slack or too tense from being held in the wrong positions and not properly exercised.

LET YOUR MIRROR BE MERCILESS

To find out literally "the shape you're in," stand in front of a full-length mirror and view yourself as critically as you would a stranger . . . front, sides and back (using a hand mirror reflection). Wear only a swim suit or nothing at all. Let your mirror be merciless in revealing the truth.

Does your head stick forward? Do your shoulders slump? Is one shoulder higher than the other? Is your upper back round? Do you have a pot-belly? Are you sway-back? Is one hip higher than the other? Does your spine curve to one side?

Analyze your posture defects and list them on a chart, with the date. Then keep a weekly record of your progress toward perfect posture . . . re-examining yourself mercilessly in the mirror each week . . . as you carry out this Fitness Program With Spine Motion. If you faithfully follow the instructions in this book, you will be highly gratified by the results, in both appearance and well-being.

BRAGG SIMPLE POSTURE EXERCISE

Here's a simple, easy way to check and reset your posture every day. Stand tall with your feet a comfortable 8-10 inches apart and your toes pointing straight forward. Put your hands on your buttocks and tighten buttocks — move hands to the lower stomach muscles, suck in stomach muscles — move hands to lower rib cage, stretch up spine and lift rib cage up — move hands to upper chest and lift chest up — move hands to shoulders and lift them up and slightly back — put right hand (second and third fingers) under chin and lift chin an inch or two — drop hands heavy by sides and swing them easily back and forth. Leave your hands swinging while you again run through the exercise.

This sets the posture naturally for you and helps you find the posture best for you. Look in the mirror to see if the shoulders are level. You may have to lift one shoulder up a little ... that will equalize them within a week.

By doing this simple exercise your body machinery will have more room to operate and your upper body will not compress the organs in your chest and abdomen. Become aware of your body mechanics!

WALKING POSTURE

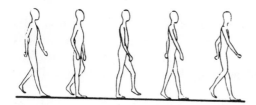

Walking posture. Always prepare a new base before leaving the old.

LIFTING POSTURE

Lifting weight. The weight of the baby is held close to the center of gravity directly above the pushing force.

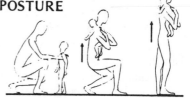

HOW TO WALK

Walking is actually a series of falls aborted by muscular force. When you realize this fact, you can better understand why it is so important to the health of your spine to walk correctly. When you "walk tall," with a full-length spine, the shock absorbers of your spinal column (cartilage plates and disks) have room to function ... and your spine acts as a spring, protecting the spinal cord and brain from the jolts of each step.

Pounding on pavements takes its toll of spinal resiliency by subjecting these natural shock absorbers to undue stress. Shoes with low rubber heels or, better still, rubber soles help to cushion the shock. Your feet are springy levers which carry the weight of your body forward with each step ... and although they need protection from hard pavements, they must not be confined or cramped but given freedom of action in well-fitted shoes. (For a thorough discussion on

30

how to fit shoes and how to develop your feet, see my book, *THE BRAGG SYSTEM OF BUILDING STRONG FEET*. To order, see back cover.)

If you have pain or discomfort in walking, the two key points to check are your feet and your spine. The Spine Motion Exercises and other stretching exercises given in this book will help greatly to make walking the buoyant, joyous exercise it is naturally supposed to be. You should swing along as though your legs began in the middle of your torso, bringing into use back, side and abdominal muscles as well as thigh, leg and foot muscles. Let your arms swing rhythmically from your shoulders ... hold your head tall and proud. Walking as Nature intended it to be is the "king" of exercise, rejuvenating the entire body.

GOOD AND BAD WAYS TO:

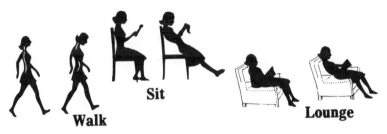

Walk **Sit** **Lounge**

HOW TO SIT PROPERLY

Slouching in a deep chair or sofa ... or slumping over a desk or table ... both distort your spine and, in different ways, put stress and strain in the wrong places ... stretching some ligaments and muscles' unduly, tensing others to compensate ... jamming some vertebrae together, pulling others out of place.

In sitting as well as standing, the same basic rules of posture apply from the hips upward, to the trunk and head ... both supported by the spine and its connecting musculoskeletal structure. The base of the spine should be at the rear of the chair seat (which should be flat and straight), the back against the chairback which should fit the natural, gentle curves of the spine. The stomach should be flat and firm, not relaxed outward ... shoulders straight, head high. In other words, "sit tall."

The flat chair seat should be shorter than the thighs, so the edge of the chair does not press against the arteries under the knees. The height

31

from seat to floor should be the length of the legs, feet flat on the floor.

Don't cross your legs! Crossing one leg over the other throws the spine out of alignment and brings on low back pain and its problems. In a woman, this unhealthy habit can cause disturbances in the female organs . . . in a man, prostate trouble.

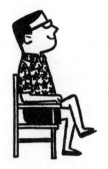

DON'T SIT WITH YOUR LEGS CROSSED!

Don't flop into a chair! Flopping into a chair, as most people do, brings extra shock to the vertebrae . . . wearing away cartilage plates and disks. Simply sitting down and rising from a chair correctly will exercise key muscles and ligaments and improve your posture. In sitting down, lower yourself into the chair lightly and gently . . . head forward and up, neck relaxed . . . spine lengthening and lower part of back widening . . . using your hip joints as hinges. Body weight is on the feet . . . ankles, legs and thighs the powerful spring levers that gently lower your body into the chair. In rising, reverse the process . . . pushing upward from your feet . . . hinging from your hips . . . spine holding head and torso in alignment. Don't use your arms to help push yourself up or lower yourself into a chair.

If you have been flopping, slouching and slumping, you may find these simple, correct methods difficult at first. But once you train yourself to sit correctly, you will find it much more relaxing and actually restful, because the body is in natural position.

KEEP YOUR SPINE ALIGNED IN BED

And speaking of restful relaxation, your spine must be in proper alignment while you are lying down . . . for a rest, a nap, or a good night's sleep. After all, we spend about one-third of our lives sleeping! And sleeping on the wrong kind of mattress can throw your spine out of alignment.

A soft, sagging mattress fails to give proper support to the heaviest part of the body, the pelvic region, and thus causes the spine to curve toward the side on which the person is sleeping. A completely rigid mattress causes the spine to curve in the opposite direction, because it does not "give" sufficiently to accommodate the wider hip and shoulder areas. Neither gives the back and spine the proper kind of support when lying on the back, or on the stomach.

A semi-rigid mattress . . . firm and flat, but with sufficient resilience to allow shoulder and pelvic bones to form their own natural hollows, keeps the spinal column in natural alignment. Placing a wide, smooth board between mattress and springs will convert any except an innerspring mattress into a semi-rigid type.

Noting that one writer has called the innerspring mattress "the devil's own work and a misbegotten gift of civilization," the well-known orthopedist, Dr. Philip Lewin, in his book on *The Back And Its Disorders* recommends a mattress of felted-cotton or hair or sponge rubber. He also advises to "stand tall" and "sit tall" and adds, "Lie tall and flat."

A small pillow, soft but firm, for your head and neck is needed to keep the upper part of your spine correctly aligned.

CHECK YOUR MATTRESS

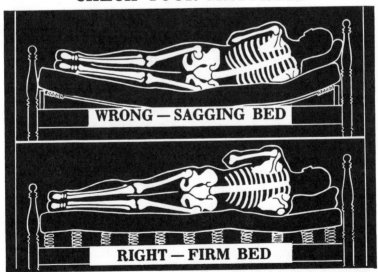

WRONG — SAGGING BED

RIGHT — FIRM BED

During sleep, you recharge the battery you ran down slowly during the day. The right kind of mattress is important. It's better to sleep ON the mattress than IN it.

Let all of your muscles be relaxed when you go to sleep. "Go limp" . . . let yourself feel "heavy" on the bed. Never let one part of the body press on the other as this will impede circulation . . . keep arms and legs apart. Tension at the back of the neck is often due to unconsciously tensed facial muscles . . . so think pleasant thoughts that make you feel like smiling.

If you have difficulty in getting sound, relaxed sleep, you will find helpful suggestions in a book of mine already mentioned, *BUILDING A POWERFUL NERVE FORCE.*

STRETCHING THE SPINE

As we noted earlier, you are "taller" when you arise in the morning, because a relaxing night's sleep allows your spinal column to stretch. Why doesn't it stay this way through the day? Why the need for special exercises?

Ordinary activities of the average person, from student to executive, housewife to movie star, simply do not utilize the spine to its full capacity. Nature constructed the human spine to withstand an enormous amount of activity, constant use and even abuse. It is this very endurance which renders the ordinary activities, and even strenuosities, inadequate in stretching the spine. Years of walking, riding, sitting, bending, turning, lifting and carrying, all have made your spinal column so accustomed to bodily exertions that it is scarcely extended to accommodate your extremities of movement.

Nature does replace to a degree the cartilage lost by constant wearing down, but there is rarely sufficient stretch of the column in modern life activities to separate the vertebrae the required amount. A little ground is lost each day . . . as is the case in Nature's restoration of tissue, blood, bone or anything else . . . and this is, essentially, what is known as the process of aging or "growing old."

Nothing, of course, can bring the process of aging to a full stop . . . but most humans accelerate it by working against Nature, failing to obey her laws. And as we have discussed, the spinal column is a key factor in practically all of our life processes. That is why Spine Motion Exercises will not only stretch your spine . . . but also stretch your life, in years and in the living of those years to the full enjoyment of vigorous health and vitality.

Animals practice natural Spine Motion. Watch a cat or dog, for example. The cat arching its back is spreading the vertebrae. A dog will

34

lower the forepart of his body, extending his forepaws far forward and writhing and twisting his head and shoulders. This natural Spine Motion is the chief reason why these animals have such unabated energy over so long a portion of their lives. A dog whose normal life is 10 years, for example, will not show any noticeable signs of ageing until his eighth or ninth year, and some will stay youthful until they are called to heaven.

We all have seen examples of people who begin to show early ageing in their 30s and 40s. But human beings were designed to stay active and energetic far longer than people might think. The human structure is mechanically adapted for full energies and activities at 70 and 80, which is clear when we see the men or women who are hale, hearty & fit, a spring in their step, clear of eye and keen of mind though well past three-quarters of a century. (see pages 78 & 79 for amazing exercise results)

Let us determine the proper leverages on the spinal column, apply them daily or every other day ... and watch premature ageing disappear. Spine Motion is so simple in application that one wonders why such a basic principle of youthfulness was so long in the discovery.

SPINE MOTION EXERCISES

To repeat, there is nothing in physiology which responds in so quick and positive a manner as the spinal column when gently but sufficiently extended to its full elastic capacity. The muscles cannot alone cause a movement ... their formation and fixed position limit the motion as well. That is why long study has been required to devise just the movements which will bring the spine into sufficient elongation ... in two different "planes" or directions ... so that the effect will be similar to the flexing given a string of beads which is turned and twisted in the hands.

Motions by which a spine is stretched must be of a character that will:
1. First of all, impose no severe strain to "rusted" positions.
2. Fall within the easy scope of the individual who has no particular development of strength.
3. Be of sufficient extremity of position to go past the mark of normal movement, be it ever so slight.

These motions have been studied to successful conclusion and achievement. They have been tested exhaustively by careful experiment and observation on hundreds of persons.

Now thousands of men and women have been benefited by the marvelous stimulus of these Spine Motion Exercises. You may be assured that the results from a very few weeks, often but a few days, of spinal elongation and torque, are so marked that one's family and friends note the difference almost as soon as the effects are inwardly felt.

SPINE MOTION BENEFITS ENTIRE BODY

Remember how, as a boy or girl, it was only parental rules for bedtime and rest that could cause you to cease activities and relax? That was because your nerves were fully insulated, protected and independent. There was a full supply of cartilage to prevent wear and tear of the longest day from impinging on any set of nerves. The spine had not started to "settle."

You can restore that condition almost 100%, at virtually any age permitting active use of the trunk muscles ... by these simple, scientific exercises which impose no hardship.

Nerves are marvelously classified and grouped. We have learned how to concentrate in the building-up process in such fashion that the vital organs can be helped separately and individually through Spine Motion ... by exercising that particular portion of the spine from which the nerves that control these organs emanate.

Numbers of people, for example, have reported that these Spine Motions, especially No. 5, have given them "magical" relief from sluggish bowels, securing perfect regularity. This is due not only to relief from pressure on the nerves, but also to the fact that the motion of the pelvis aids elimination by making the large intestine twist and coil about and squeeze at the sharper turns where waste is so apt to accumulate.

There are many such "bonuses" that come from these Spine Motion Exercises. By scientifically stretching your spine, you will at the same time strengthen the muscles and ligaments that support it ... thus helping to hold the elongation ... and greatly improving your posture. Circulation and nerve energy will be stimulated throughout your body. Digestion will improve, as pressure on controlling nerves is relieved ... and as organs become more firmly supported in correct position. You will find that you are breathing more deeply ... giving your body cells more of that priceless "invisible food," oxygen.

36

MAKE EVERY MOTION COUNT

It is essential to put "form" into the performance of these exercises. The entire set of motions will not consume a consequential amount of time . . . nor will they cause more than momentary fatigue. So don't "slide through" them. Just as the routine movements of daily living are inadequate in keeping the spine limber and long . . . so a perfunctory performance of even these special movements cannot be expected to produce the desired results.

You must throw a full measure of energy and enthusiasm into these Spine Motion Exercises. But don't overdo! For the first week or so, do the exercises slowly . . . feel your way, stopping short of the point of pain or fatigue. You will find this point extending day by day, as nervous energy is released and muscles strengthen.

When you first start limbering up the back, you may have some muscle soreness . . . but don't stop exercising. After a few days of continuous daily periods of exercise, the muscle soreness will disappear. Soon you will find great satisfaction in doing these spinal exercises . . . and the beneficial effects will amaze you.

Now, let's get started! There are five main Spine Motion Exercises . . . each different in effect, though similar in general aspects. Take a momentary rest between each one . . . but do the entire series.

SPINE MOTION EXERCISE NO. 1

This first Spine Motion specifically applies to nerves which affect the head and the eye muscles. A reflex of the same motion affects a set of nerves that go to the stomach and bowels. Thus in one movement, we attack the cause of headaches, eye strain, indigestion and poor assimilation.

Lie face down on the floor. Now, raise to an arched position in which you rest on hands and toes with the back highly arched. (See Figure 1, Position 1.) The pelvis will be higher than the head. Feet are spread about 15 inches apart. Knees and elbows must be kept stiff.

Now, drop the pelvis almost to the floor. (See Figure 1, Position 2.) Remember, elbows and knees stiff . . . this is essential to impart the proper spinal stretch. As you lower the back, throw your head back . . . raise it sharply as you lower the body.

This is not a fast motion . . . take time in its execution. Dip to the extreme low limit . . . raise high again, arching the back all you can . . .

down again ... up ... and down. If you do this motion correctly, you will find that a very few times seem "enough." If only some way could be devised for you to see what is going on along the spinal column during this jackknife action, you would know the relaxation and relief imparted to the nerves all along the line.

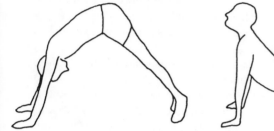

FIGURE No.1 - POSITION 1

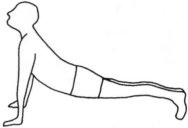

FIGURE No.1 - POSITION 2

SPINE MOTION EXERCISE NO. 2

This second Spine Motion is designed particularly to stimulate the nerves leading to the liver and kidneys. It brings relief from a score of nervous conditions which are manifested in subnormal functioning of these vital organs. A sluggish liver and non-elastic kidneys ... prematurely "aged," for which there is no real excuse ... will respond with surprising swiftness to spinal torque or twist. This second motion will bring these organs quickly to a state of vigorous function.

This motion starts in the same arched position as No. 1. (See Figure 1, Position 1.) Face down, weight resting on hands and toes, back highly arched, elbows and knees stiff.

Now, swing the pelvis slowly from one side to the other ... to the very limit of your ability in each move to the right, then to the left ... back and forth. (See Figure 2, Position 2.) This motion should be done slowly. Think always of the s-t-r-e-t-c-h we must give the spinal column.

You will find this motion tiring at first. It will grow constantly easier to do ... not because of muscular development so much as because of vastly improved nervous organization. But it should never become perfectly easy. This is more than a simple swaying of your body ... you must make every one of the long row of vertebrae pull away from those adjoining it.

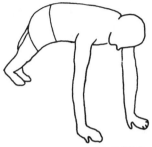

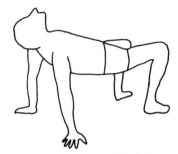

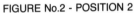

FIGURE No.2 - POSITION 2   FIGURE No.3 - POSITION 3

SPINE MOTION EXERCISE NO. 3

In this third Spine Motion the entire spinal column is flexed from top to base. Every nerve center is stimulated. The pelvic region is specifically helped. This motion also strengthens those muscles attached to the spine which are most helpful in retaining the vertebrae in improved, elongated position ... stimulating the growth of inter-vertebral cartilage.

Take a new starting position for this motion. Sit down on the floor ... then raise the pelvis by placing hands at sides (palms down) and drawing in the feet about 12 inches. You are now resting your weight on the flat of the hands and the feet, the pelvis just off the floor.

This motion is rapid. Raise the body rapidly ... let the spine be horizontal as you finish the upward movement. (See Figure 3, Position 3.) Now, down rapidly to the starting position ... lowering yourself to the point which just misses the floor ... up once more ... down ... etc. A very fast motion is required here. Its benefits are marked.

SPINE MOTION EXERCISE NO. 4

The fourth Spine Motion brings particular force to bear at the curve of the spine where nerves affecting the stomach are clustered. This motion also has the greatest efficiency of the whole series in the actual lengthening of the spine from tip to tip ... and the results are felt in overall general improvement. After all, it is the general stretching of the entire spinal column which brings the whole system to balanced efficacy.

Lie on the floor on your back, hands at sides. Bend the knees and bring to chest position ... clasping arms around the legs a few inches below the knees. Now pull knees and thighs tightly against chest. At the same time raise the head and try to touch the chin to the knees. (See Figure 4, Position 4.) Hold this squeezing position at least five seconds.

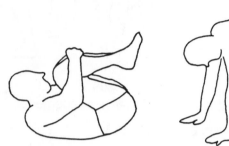

FIGURE No.4 - POSITION 4

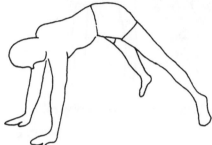

FIGURE No.5 - POSITION 5

SPINE MOTION EXERCISE NO. 5

In addition to its spine stretching benefits, this fifth Spine Motion is the one previously referred to, which brings such speedy relief to sluggish bowels both by nerve stimulation and corollary exercise to the large intestine.

Again assume Position No. 1 ... by lying face down on the floor ... then raising to an arched position, resting on hands and toes ... the back highly arched, pelvis higher than the head. (See Figure 5, Position 5.) Now walk all around the room in this all-fours position.

HOW MANY TIMES AND HOW OFTEN?

The number of times for each of these Spine Motion Exercises will rest with the individual. At first, 3 to 5 times for each Spine Motion will extend you amply. In a day or two increase the count to 5 times, or more. Since these motions are entirely new, you will experience muscular stiffness during the first few days ... but this will pass. After the period of stiffness, when spine and muscles and ligaments become
(cont. on page 43)

Leg cramps often indicate circulatory problems and show that you need more exercise, walking, stretching, good posture and deep breathing. It also indicates that you need to take a multi mineral-vitamin supplement with ample magnesium, calcium and all the balance of minerals, including trace minerals — boron, etc. — and Vitamins E, C, A, B-Complex with extra B-12 and niacin. These all add up to good basic insurance for more super health. Also alternating hot then cold foot & calf baths help increase circulation.

Reflexology, or Zone Therapy — Founded by Eunice Ingham, author of "The Story The Feet Can Tell," whose health career was inspired by a Bragg Health Crusade when she was 17. Relieves the body by removing crystalline deposits from meridians (nerve endings) of the feet by using deep pressure massage. A form of Reflexology massage has its early origins in China and is known to have been practiced by Kenyan natives and North American Indian tribes for centuries. Treatment is a firm pressure stroking along the pressure points in the feet by the therapist's fingers.

Reiki — A Japanese form of massage which means "Universal Life Energy." Life energy radiates from the hands of a Reiki therapist. It was discovered in the ancient Sutra manuscripts by Dr. Mikso Usui.

Rolfing — This technique was developed by Ida Rolf in the 1930s in the U.S., and is sometimes called structural processing, postural release or structural dynamics. It is based on the concept that distortions of nominal function of organs and skeletal muscles occur throughout life, and are accentuated by the effects of gravity on the body. Rolfing methods help the individual to achieve balance and improved body posture. Methods involve the use of stretching, deep tissue massage and relaxation techniques to loosen old injuries and break bad movement patterns which cause long-term body stress.

Self Massage — Paul Bragg often said, "You can be your own best masseuse, even if you have only one good hand." Near-miraculous improvements have been achieved by victims of accidents or strokes in bringing life back to afflicted parts of their own bodies by self-massage and even vibrators. Treatments can be day or night, almost continual. Also, self-massage can help achieve relaxation at day's end. Families and friends can exchange massages; it's a wonderful sharing experience. Remember, babies love massages.

Aromatic Massage — It works two ways: The essence (smell) helps the patient relax as does the massage itself, while the massage is used to help absorption of essential natural oils used for centuries to treat numerous complaints. For example, Tiger Balm helps relieve muscle aches. Avoid creams and lotions with mineral oil because it clogs pores. Almond, olive, peanut and grape seed oil are among the most popular. There are 30-40 aromatics to use derived from herbs and other botanicals. Pure rosemary oil — 6 drops to 6 ounces of almond oil — is a favorite.

(Continued on page 42)

Shiatsu — It means "finger pressure" in Japanese and is applied with pressure from the fingers, hands, elbows and even knees along the same 12 meridian paths used in acupuncture, which was used for centuries in the Orient to relieve pain, common ills and muscle stress and to aid lymphatic circulation.

Sports Massage — Developed over the years into a sophisticated, important support system for athletes, professional and amateur. Sports massage serves these functions, according to an AMTA brochure: improving circulation and mobility to injured tissue, enabling the athlete to recover more rapidly from myofascial injury, reducing muscle soreness and chronic strain patterns. Soft tissues are freed of trigger points and adhesions, thus contributing toward improvement of peak neuromuscular functioning and athletic performance. It's a preventive approach to injuries that can be suffered during training and it provides a psychological boost to the athlete.

Tragering — Founded by Dr. Milton Trager M.D., who was inspired at age 18 by Paul Bragg to study health. It is an experimental learning method which involves gentle shaking and rocking, suggesting a greater letting go, releasing and lengthening of muscles for body health. Tragering can do miraculous healing where needed in the muscles and entire body.

Water Therapy — Showers are wonderful. First apply olive oil to skin, then hot and cold shower and massage needed areas while under shower. Tub baths are wonderful as well: Apply oil and massage. You can add Epsom salts if your muscles ache or 1 cup of apple cider vinegar. Try dry skin light-brushing — it's wonderful for circulation, toning and healing. Also for variety use a loofah sponge for massaging in the shower and tub.

Swedish Massage — Oldest and most-used massage technique. Deep body massage that soothes, promotes circulation and is also a great way to loosen muscles before and after exercise.

Author's Comment: I have personally sampled all of these techniques, as did my father. Many of the founders were our personal friends. It has made it all the more enjoyable to know how and why they started their health outreach, living lives of service and promoting wellness! In an age where everyone wants health and youthfulness, more and more new styles of massage are becoming popular. My advice to readers: "Seek and find the best for your body, mind, and spirit."

– Patricia Bragg

(cont. from page 40)
more limber, a normally strong person (man or woman) will find 10 times for each exercise no more difficult than were the 3 times of the first day.

How long should you continue this series of Spine Motion Exercises? In the beginning, your spine stretching routine should be a regular daily program. After you show marked improvement, twice weekly is usually sufficient to keep the spine flexed.

Some people report that the very first session with Spine Motion Exercises has brought every apparent benefit promised ... but it usually requires a week to see and feel the change. It is two or three weeks before the ground gained begins to take hold organically and assumes permanence of effect.

Please bear in mind that the settling process of the spine has been a matter of years. It is not a condition you can overcome in a day ... but a single execution of the movements does give the spine time to stay stretched and stimulate cartilage growth. Faithful daily practice of these exercises allows quick growth of cartilage under favorable conditions ... thus securing the widened spaces between the vertebrae.

SPINE STRENGTHENING EXERCISES

In addition to the unique Bragg Spine Motion Exercises, some of the basic physical therapy exercises recommended by many orthopedists are excellent for strengthening the spine and its supporting muscles. I have selected a dozen of these for inclusion in this Fitness Program, as follows:

No. 1 ... **Neck Extension for Strengthening Upper Spine.** Stand in correct posture position, feet slightly apart, muscles relaxed. Clasp hands behind your head. Lean your head forward, then attempt to push it backward as you resist with your hands. Do this for 6 seconds ... counting one-thousand-and-one, one-thousand-and-two, etc. Repeat with head straight up ... then with head as far back as possible. Stretch your neck as far as you can in each direction.

No. 2 ... **Back Strengthening and Stretching.** This exercise will give wonderful relief whenever your back feels tired. Stand up and stretch, feet slightly apart, rising on your toes and reaching upward with arms ... then relax. Now bend over at the waist, knees slightly bent. Hold your legs with your hands behind the knees. Pull in your stomach muscles and attempt to straighten your back, while resisting back extension with your hands. Hold for 6 seconds ... counting one-

thousand-and-one, one-thousand-and-two, etc. Then relax . . .
stretch . . . relax. Feel better?

No. 3 . . . Leg Extension for Strengthening Back. Lean over a table,
palms of hands flat on top near the edge, elbows bent . . . standing far
enough away so that head and torso bend comfortably parallel to table
top, spine straight. Keep knees stiff, feet flat on floor. Now slowly raise
one leg backward as high as possible. Hold for 6 seconds . . . counting
one-thousand-and-one, etc. Slowly lower leg to starting position.
Repeat with other leg. Continue, alternating legs, but stop when you
begin to tire.

No. 4 . . . Neck Rolling to Strengthen Upper Spine. Stand in a
comfortable correct posture position with no tension. Now bring your
chin to your chest . . . roll your head to one side, trying to make your
ear touch your shoulder . . . continue roll toward your back, stretching
the neck as far backward as possible . . . rolling on to the other side,
trying to touch that shoulder with that ear . . . then rolling head back
to starting position. Do this exercise slowly, s-t-r-e-t-c-h-i-n-g the neck
muscles . . . 20 times from right to left, 20 times from left to right. This
exercise is a "must" for desk workers to relieve muscular tension in the
neck and keep the cervical vertebrae properly extended.

No. 5 . . . Rag Doll Exercise for Strengthening Entire Spine. Stand in
comfortable correct posture position, feet about 18 inches apart.
Pretend your arms are those of a rag doll, completely limp . . . letting
them bounce limply as you swing your body from one side to the
other . . . turning with each swing to look as far back as you can over
each shoulder.

No. 6 . . . The "Old Favorite" Spine Exercise. Stand erect with feet
together. Raise hands over head, arms straight. Keeping the knees stiff,
bend forward and try to touch your toes with your fingertips. Bounce
your torso downward to reach as far as possible. Return to starting
position. Then, with arms upraised, bend backward as far as possible,
dropping head and arms backward. Return to starting position. Repeat
at least 10 times.

No. 7 . . . Spinal Twisting Exercise. Stand in correct posture position, feet about 18 inches apart. Extend arms to shoulder height at
sides. Holding arms in position, twist your body from the hips as far as
possible to the right, letting your eyes follow the back of the right
hand . . . then as far as possible to the left. Try to see the same thing
directly in back of you when you twist to each side. Alternating from
right to left, repeat this exercise 30 times.

No. 8 . . . Endurance Test to Strengthen Lower Spine. Lie flat on your back on the floor, arms at sides. Keeping the knees stiff, lift your heels two inches off the floor . . . and try to hold your legs and feet off the floor in this position for 60 seconds . . . counting one-thousand-and-one, etc. Each time you do this exercise add a few more seconds. This really gives the lower spine a wonderful workout.

No. 9 . . . Hip Rolling Exercise for Strengthening Lower Spine. Lie flat on your back on the floor, arms extended at sides at shoulder height, feet together. Raise the right leg vertically, toes pointed upward, knee straight . . . then swing it to the left, touching toes to floor beyond fingertips of left hand. Return leg to vertical position, then lower it to floor. Repeat same exercise with left leg beyond fingertips of right hand. Do this exercise 20 times, alternating right and left legs.

No. 10 . . . On-the-Side Exercise for Strengthening Entire Spine. Lie on the floor on your right side, legs straight, arms comfortable. Keeping the knee stiff, raise your left leg straight up . . . then return it slowly to starting position. Now bend the knee and bring your left thigh up against your chest . . . and try to touch your chin to the knee. Do this exercise 10 times on the right side . . . then turn over to the left side and repeat 10 times with the right leg.

No. 11 . . . Arm-Hanging Spine-Stretcher. If you have or have access to wall bars, do this exercise from a rung high enough for your feet to clear the floor. If not, use a door which is fully open and steady so it cannot swing, and place a towel over the top edge so you can get a good grip. Now grasp the top of the door (or rung of wall bars) and relax your body, letting it hang free. If you use a door, bend your knees so your feet will be off the floor. Remember, this is an exercise for your back, not your arms, so make your body dead-weight to s-t-r-e-t-c-h your spine. Hang like this as long as you can, then relax briefly and do it again, and again . . . at least three times.

No. 12 . . . The Shoulder-Shrug for Cervical Vertebrae. Stand in correct posture position, feet together or slightly apart. Roll your shoulders up as far as possible . . . forward as far as possible . . . and back as far as possible . . . in a smooth, continuous motion. Do this 15 times. Pause briefly, then reverse the rotation for 15 times . . . up . . . back . . . forward. Increase daily from 15 to 30 times each way.

We are all manufacturers, making goods,
making trouble or making excuses.

EXERCISE THROUGHOUT THE DAY

The first seven of these Spine Strengthening Exercises can be done anywhere, anytime. Sedentary workers especially . . . from typist to executive . . . should get up from time to time, stretch, and do at least one of these exercises. You will return to your work refreshed and with renewed energy . . . instead of losing time, you will save it because you will be able to work faster and better after a genuine exercise "breather." And you will save your health, too!

Dr. Henry L. Feffer, professor of orthopedic surgery at the George Washington University School of Medicine, noted in a recent interview that the greatest strain on the intervertebral disks occurs while sitting, "especially in an overstuffed chair."

"The pressure per square inch on a disk is about twice as great when sitting as when standing," he said. "And this pressure is more likely to injure a disk if it does not have a good external muscular support—which is often the case in a sedentary person."

Dr. Feffer also commented, "Usually the chair that an office executive gives his stenographer is a much better chair for the back than the swivel chair he uses himself."

So . . . if you are a sedentary worker, as the great majority of Americans are . . . be sure you use a chair that helps you to maintain correct posture at all times . . . and be sure to get up out of that chair (correctly!) at intervals to stretch your spinal column and strengthen your muscles.

Get off the elevator several floors below your own and walk up the final flights of stairs . . . head and chest up, spine in perfect alignment. Don't pull yourself up by the handrail . . . push yourself from one stairstep to the next by the springy leverage of your foot.

Even if your work involves physical labor . . . remember that it is not necessarily the amount of exercise you do . . . but the way you do it that counts. Remember the case of the lumberjack who "chopped" his spine out of alignment! If the muscles on one side of your spinal column are developed more than on the other, the spine can be pulled into a side curvature. Take time for exercises that "balance" those required in your work.

If your daily activities are primarily those of running a household, you will find that your everyday duties will become much easier and less fatiguing if you utilize some of the movements given in these strengthening and stretching exercises in your work . . . and also take "breathers" at intervals to stretch your spine and strengthen unused muscles.

And since most schools today do not require regular "physical ed," teenagers and college students . . . who have "outgrown" vigorous childhood games and recreation . . . need to make a daily habit of spine stretching and strengthening exercises. Spines can begin to "settle" even in your teens!

THE "DOG STRETCH" EXERCISE

Among the orthopedic exercises recommended by Dr. Arthur A. Michele, chairman of orthopedic surgery at New York Medical College and director of orthopedic surgery at eight other New York City hospitals, in his recent book on *Orthotherapy,* is a spine-stretcher which I think deserves special attention. Although Dr. Michele calls it the "Long Body Stretch," I call it the "Dog Stretch," because it reminds me of the dog's natural Spine Motion previously referred to.

Kneel on the floor with your knees 6 to 8 inches apart. Keeping your thighs perpendicular to the floor, bend forward from the waist . . . stretching your arms forward along the floor until your forehead touches the floor . . . your torso sloping down from hips to elbows.

Now lower your chest as close to the floor as you can . . . pressing down for a fast count of ten. Return to starting (sloping) position for a count of five. Repeat as many times as you can in 3 minutes.

This exercise stretches the entire spine as well as limbering the shoulder joints.

We have all seen animals, from rabbits to horses, lie on their backs and wiggle their backbones in the soil. According to another orthopedist, Dr. Lloyd Kingsbery, they are not merely scratching their backs . . . they are exercising their spines. He adapted this exercise to humans as follows:

Lie on your back, knees bent, feet about 18 inches apart . . . arms extended on floor at shoulder height, elbows bent with forearms parallel to head. Press the small of your back (lumbar vertebrae) flat against the floor . . . inching your hips downward and your shoulders and head upward as your spine stretches. Hold your body in this "natural traction" position as long as possible, relaxing when your muscles begin to tire.

Whether you feel tired or your back aches from physical or sedentary labor, these two exercises give wonderful, spine-stretching relief.

OVERWEIGHT OVERLOADS YOUR SPINE

When you consider that 1300 pounds of pull are exerted on your spine and sacroiliac joints simply to maintain an erect posture . . . and that practically the entire weight of your vital organs is borne by the spine . . . you can understand why an excess burden of fat usually results in chronic backache. As we have discussed, your spine has enough jobs to do without having to carry a needless overload. I am sure you would rebel if you were forced to wear a sack filled with ten to a hundred pounds of rocks suspended from your waist at all times. Yet that is exactly the kind of overload you force upon your spine when you are overweight.

Overweight exacts other penalties, too. It overburdens the heart, not only with fatty tissue around this muscular organ, but by forcing it to strain and overwork in pumping blood through the additional miles of blood vessels. High blood pressure often develops. Fat deposits on other vital organs, such as the kidneys and pancreas, impedes their functioning.

Dr. Lewin, whom I have quoted previously, states in *The Back And Its Disorders:*

"Persons are too much inclined to laugh off overweight and to dismiss it lightly. Doctors, however, regard it as a disease, and an insidious one at that. It is particularly treacherous because the fat person may *feel* fit as a fiddle for a long time. But he can depend on it that his years will be decreased in direct ratio to the number of extra pounds of fat he carries.

"The back is directly affected by overweight, and as a preventive, as well as a curative, measure, anyone who has back troubles or who wishes to avoid them should watch those bathroom scales. After the age of thirty-five, everyone is better off when he's a few pounds underweight."

Massage helps in soothing, releasing, and making you aware of the body. The trained "touch-skilled" therapist using their hands and fingers as a diagnostic tool can feel them. Some are the size of tiny peas and toxic wastes often get locked up in these knotted muscles, connective tissues and sore, injured areas. A good therapist has in their hands the ability to help the body flush out these toxic wastes and restore more health to the tissues by releasing these toxins! Remember the body is self-repairing and self-healing when given the opportunity! Massages are good health aids!

A REGIMEN FOR REDUCING

If you are overweight, don't delude yourself that there is a "quick cure." I have had many people complain to me that they have tried this and that "crash diet" ... or one or another "sure way to reduce with dieting" ... without any lasting benefit. They have suffered various discomforts for short periods losing a certain number of pounds ... only to regain this lost weight, and sometimes more, as soon as the "crash course" was over.

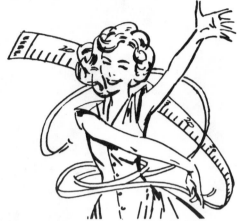

In my more than 65 years as nutritionist and physical conditioner, I have helped thousands of men and women to attain and maintain healthy, normal weight by natural methods. I know of no other way to accomplish permanent weight control than by making it a way of life ... establishing a regular regimen of diet and exercise that keeps your metabolism in proper balance. Metabolism is the intricate process by which your body converts food into energy. When you take in more fuel (food) than you burn up in energy (activities), the excess is stored as fat.

A thorough treatment of the subject of losing weight and maintaining it at normal level is given in my book, *THE NATURAL WAY TO REDUCE*. (See back cover for ordering.) This program has been successfully followed by many stars in the theatrical and athletic worlds, as well as numerous other health students around the globe. If you are ten pounds or more overweight ... or if you are developing a tendency in this direction ... this book will prove a valuable addition to your Health Library.

Famous Comedian & Author Dick Gregory weighed 320 pounds and his inspiration was our Miracle of Fasting book that guided him into healthy lifestyle living that was life-changing for him. He traded his bad habits – dead, processed foods, drinking, drugs, smoking, etc for healthy habits!!! He now weighs a trim, fit 150 pounds and has been in eight Boston Marathons. He is now guiding others to reduce and live on live foods and abstain from unnatural, processed foods. Dick praises our Building Powerful Nerve Force book also – as he said he now has nerves of steel - thanks to our teachings in that mighty little book.

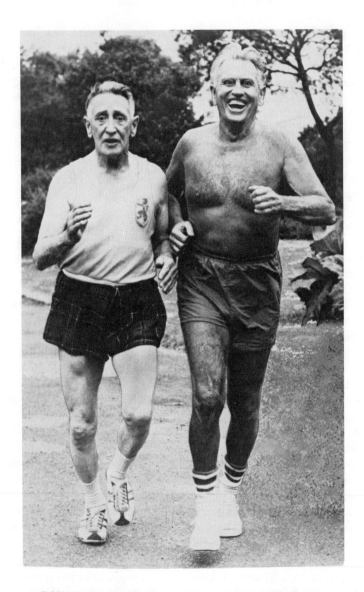

DUNCAN MCLEAN AND PAUL C. BRAGG
England's oldest Champion Sprinter (**93** years young) on a training jog in London's famous Regent's Park. They keep their spines youthful and flexible by exercise and right diet.

NATURAL DIET AND NATURAL WEIGHT

One reason that overweight is such a prevalent problem today . . . in every age group . . . is that most people eat the wrong kind of food and too much. In connection with overeating, Dr. Lewin makes this pithy comment:

". . . Two exercises, especially, are most beneficial to the reducer. The first is a shaking of the head from side to side when second helpings are passed, and the second is a pushing movement away from the table while still hungry!"

Let me add that these maxims apply not only to the reducer, but also to everyone in maintaining a normal, natural weight. I have never had an extra ounce of flesh on my body . . . and I have always made it a rule to get up from the table while still feeling a little bit hungry. The result is that I never feel sluggish, and am always full of energy and vitality.

Another succinct piece of advice from Dr. Lewin, which I have also preached and practiced throughout a long, healthy lifetime, is:

". . . A good reducing diet, one recommended by a physician, gives the reducer all the necessary vitamins, minerals, and proteins necessary to his body's health. When there is any chance that the essential food elements may not be ingested in sufficient quantities in the food, additional food elements are prescribed in capsule or tablet form."

This is from an orthopedist speaking particularly to patients whose backaches are due primarily to excess fat. But again let me say that it is sound advice for everyone.

A diet of natural foods is the surest way to maintain natural weight as well as good health. In Mother Nature's design for living, she has provided perfectly balanced nutrition for every living thing in both the plant and animal kingdoms.

Man, however, in attempting to redesign this pattern to his own convenience, has upset this balance . . . and is paying the penalty in loss of health. Our industrialized civilization has concentrated masses of people in centers distant from their sources of natural food supply. The resulting necessity for mass transportation, storage and distribution of foodstuffs has transformed the average diet into an artificial one . . . made up primarily of devitalized, demineralized, devitamized, processed, additive-ridden "dead" foods . . . which may seem to satisfy the demands of hunger but do not satisfy the natural demands of the body. In the last 50 years the American diet has deteriorated to such an extent that our children walk around with little energy, flabby fat, and weak, slumped spines. In a desperate effort to get a "lift," many of them resort to drugs. So do adults . . . from coffee and tea, alcohol and nicotine, the slow killers . . . to those which are more speedily fatal.

Is it possible to live on a natural diet in this polluted world? Yes, it is! It requires a certain amount of effort and discrimination . . . but the rewards are great. Isn't it worth a little effort to exchange the misery of mere existence for the joy of vital, glowing, healthy life?

ELIMINATE "DEAD" FOODS FROM YOUR DIET

When man discovered that salt kept meat from spoiling, he added the first preservative . . . and the first poison . . . to his natural food. This happened so long ago that the majority of people have long thought of salt as a natural human food. It isn't! It is an inorganic, indigestible mineral, sodium chloride . . . not to be confused with pure organic sodium, which the human body assimilates and needs. Sodium

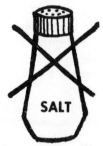

chloride, common table salt, has no nutritive value whatever. The human body eliminates as much of it as possible . . . and stores the residue in water solution in bodily tissue, often with disastrous results. Today, the harmful effects of salt . . . still the most widely used food preservative . . . are aggravated by a host of new chemical preservatives and additives which are also poisonous.

The other major crime against natural foods has come about through refining or processing. Refined white flour has a long "shelf life" because it is actually "dead" . . . the vital raw wheat germ, one of Nature's richest sources of nutrition, having been refined out of it, leaving nothing but empty calories. The same sort of thing has happened to sugar . . . the essential enzymes and vitamins eliminated by the refining process. The energy content of refined white sugar as compared to pure raw sugar is like the burning of a sheet of newspaper compared to a steady wood fire.

In a similar manner processed meats and cheeses have been completely devitalized. Hydrogenated oils and margarines have been hardened into indigestible, insoluble lumps of waxy fat.

So . . . for your health and your life . . . take your glasses (if you need them) to market with you and read the food labels! Eliminate the dead, embalmed foodstuffs from your diet! Here is a guide list:

52

AVOID THESE PROCESSED, REFINED, HARMFUL FOODS

Once you realize the irreparable harm caused to your body by refined, chemicalized, deficient foods, it is not difficult to eat correctly. Simply eliminate these "killer" foods from your diet...and follow an eating plan which provides the basic, essential nourishment your body needs.

- Refined sugar or refined sugar products such as jams, jellies, preserves, marmalades, yogurts, ice cream, sherberts, Jello, cake, candy, cookies, chewing gum, soft drinks, pies, pastries, tapioca puddings, sugared fruit juices & fruits canned in sugar syrup.

- Salted foods, such as corn chips, salted crackers, salted nuts

- Catsup & mustard w/salt-sugar, Worchestershire sauce, pickles, olives

- White rice & pearled barley   • Fried & greasy foods

- Commercial, highly processed dry cereals such as corn flakes, etc.

- Saturated fats & hydrogenated oils...(heart enemies that clog bloodstream)

- Food which contains palm & cottonseed oil. Products labeled vegetable oil...find out what kind, before you use it.

- Oleo & margarines...(saturated fats & hydrogenated oils)

- Peanut butter that contains hydrogenated, hardened oils

- Coffee, decaffeinated coffee, China black tea & all alcoholic beverages

- Fresh pork & pork products   • Fried, fatty & greasy meats

- Smoked meats, such as ham, bacon & sausage, smoked fish

- Luncheon meats, such as hot dogs, salami, bologna, corned beef, pastrami & any packaged meats containing dangerous sodium nitrate or nitrite

- Dried fruits containing sulphur dioxide - a preservative

- Do not eat chickens that have been injected with stilbestrol, or fed with chicken feed that contains any drug

- Canned soups - read labels for sugar, starch, white, wheat flour & preservatives

- Food that contains benzoate of soda, salt, sugar, cream of tartar...& any additives, drugs or preservatives

- White flour products such as white bread, wheat-white bread, enriched flours, rye bread that has wheat-white flour in it, dumplings, biscuits, buns, gravy, noodles, pancakes, waffles, soda crackers, macaroni, spaghetti, pizza, ravioli, pies, pastries, cakes, cookies , prepared and commercial puddings, and ready-mix bakery products. (Health Stores have a huge variety of 100% whole grain products.)

- Day-old, cooked vegetables & potatoes, & pre-mixed old salads

FOOD AND PRODUCT SUMMARY

Today many of our foods are highly processed or refined, thus robbing them of essential nutrients, vitamins, minerals, and enzymes; many contain harmful and dangerous chemicals.

The research, findings, and experience of top nutritionists, physicians and dentists have led them to discover that devitalized foods are a major cause of poor health, illness, cancer and premature death. The enormous increase in the last seventy years in degenerative diseases such as heart disease, arthritis, and dental decay, would seem to substantiate this belief. Scientific research has shown most of these afflictions may be prevented; and others, when once established, may be arrested or in some cases even reversed through nutritional methods.

THESE STEPS ARE FOR SUPER HEALTH THROUGH HEALTHY, WHOLESOME, NATURAL FOOD

1. Serve foods in raw, original state, organically grown when possible – fresh fruits, vegetables, wholegrains, brown rice, beans, raw nuts & seeds.

2. PROTEIN

    a. Animal meat, including the variety meats — liver, kidney, brain, heart — poultry and sea food, suggest using sparingly. Cook meat as little as possible (bake, roast, wok, or broil) because protein is injured by prolonged high heat. (My Dad and I prefer a vegetarian diet.)

    b. Dairy products, eggs (fertile), unprocessed hard cheese, and certified raw milk. (Personally we do not use milk and only occasionally low-fat dairy by-products).

    c. The legumes, soy and all other beans ... these are our favorites.

    d. Nuts and seeds, raw and unsalted.

3. Use FRUITS and VEGETABLES (organically grown without the use of poisonous chemical sprays and fertilizers, when possible). Ask your market to stock organic produce. Steam, bake, saute or wok vegetables with a minimum of distilled water, at low heat, for as short a time as possible. Use the vegetable liquid.

4. Use 100% WHOLEGRAIN CEREALS, BREADS, & FLOURS, they contain important B complex vitamins, vitamin E, minerals, & the important unsaturated fatty acids.

5. Use COLD-PROCESSED VEGETABLE OILS, OLIVE OIL, CANOLA and SESAME OIL, etc.... These are an excellent source of the healthy essential unsaturated fatty acids, but still use sparingly.

4 BRAGG BOOKS FOR PLANNING HEALTHY MEALS

These Books are a must reading for planning your Bragg Health Building Program. They are: • *Healthful Eating Without Confusion* • *Bragg's Health Gourmet Recipes For Vital Healthy Living* (448 pages) • *Bragg Vegetarian Health Gourmet Recipes* (sugar free, salt free, low fat) and the • *Bragg Health Sauerkraut (raw, salt free) Recipe Book* ... Learn why and how to make your own delicious sauerkraut – it's so healthy for you. See back pages for ordering.

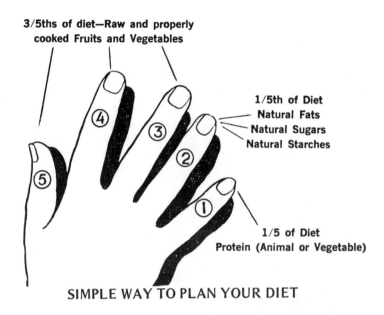

3/5ths of diet—Raw and properly cooked Fruits and Vegetables

④ ③ ② ⑤ ①

**1/5th of Diet
Natural Fats
Natural Sugars
Natural Starches**

**1/5 of Diet
Protein (Animal or Vegetable)**

SIMPLE WAY TO PLAN YOUR DIET

1. Fresh Fruits and Vegetables should comprise Three-Fifths of Your Diet ... This includes raw fresh fruit and vegetables and their juices and properly cooked vegetables. By juices I mean freshly squeezed in a juicer or blender, not canned or frozen.

The ideal way to start your day is with FRESH FRUIT or fruit juice. It is also the perfect dessert for any meal ... and the only between-meal snack you should ever take. For dessert you may also have sun-dried fruits, which are best when soaked overnight in distilled water.

Your midday and evening meals should always begin with a SALAD OF FRESH, RAW VEGETABLES. And please get out of the rut of considering tomatoes and lettuce to be the only salad ingredients! There is nothing more delicious and nutritious for lunch than a large mixed vegetable salad ... combining green lettuce, finely chopped green celery, grated carrots, grated raw beets, sliced cucumbers (skin included), radishes, parsley, watercress, green onions, diced green peppers and sliced tomatoes ... or various combinations of these ingredients. If an avocado is available, chop it into the salad. Use a lemon and oil dressing with a dash of natural cider vinegar, and season with powdered kelp. Raw cabbage also makes a wonderful salad base and is rich in Vitality Vitamin C, so important for the health of your spine and other bones. Salt-free sauerkraut, which you can make at home, makes a wonderful topping. (See back pages regarding my *SALT-FREE HEALTH SAUERKRAUT COOK BOOK*)

PROPERLY COOKED VEGETABLES are also important in a balanced diet. Cook your vegetables as soon after buying or picking as possible . . . and don't overcook! Many valuable vitamins are lost by overcooking and also by peeling. Wash vegetables thoroughly and cook them in their skins . . . either baked, or over low heat in the least amount of water necessary. Pressure cooking and steam cooking are excellent methods.

2. Proteins should constitute One-Fifth of Your Diet . . . These may be either animal or vegetable or a mixture of both.

ANIMAL PROTEINS include meat, fish, poultry, eggs, milk and natural cheese. In selecting meat and poultry, be sure these are from an uncontaminated source . . . free from stilbestrol or other harmful drugs. And make sure that your fish is from non-mercury waters. Because of the uric acid content in meat, I recommend limiting meat in your menus to three times per week. And don't forget organ meats . . . heart, kidneys, etc. . . . contain much higher nutritional values than muscle meat, as well as being less expensive. Eggs should be fresh and fertile, from 4 to 6 per week in the average diet. Pure, natural cheeses . . . natural cheddar and other raw natural cheeses, and yoghurt . . . are an excellent source of protein and combine well with salads, as well as casserole dishes. Milk . . . whole milk, raw or certified . . . is a fine protein source for growing children, but not as well assimilated by adults. The same is true of buttermilk. Milk and its products can often cause mucus and other problems for some people—if so—eliminate from your diet.

VEGETABLE PROTEINS include soy beans, dried beans such as kidney, pinto and lima, lentils and garbanzos . . . avocado, raw nuts and seeds, nut butter and sesame seed butter . . . whole grains such as barley, buckwheat, corn, millet and wheat . . . raw wheat germ and brewer's yeast . . . eggplant and mushrooms . . . and alfalfa sprouts, which are as excellent a source of vegetable protein as you can find and which you can grow easily indoors. Raw wheat germ is also one of the richest natural sources of versatile Vitamin E and other important nutrients . . . and adds zest when sprinkled over whole grain cereals and salads.

56

A wide variety of delicious entrees can be made from vegetable proteins, and I have known many wonderfully healthy people who were strict vegetarians. Others prefer a lacto-vegetarian diet, getting their proteins from dairy products and vegetables . . . while others, like myself, enjoy and thrive on a combination of animal and vegetable proteins. It is up to you to choose what suits you best . . . just so you make sure that one-fifth of your daily diet is protein, the body's "building blocks."

3. Natural Fats, Starches and Sugars make up the final One-Fifth of Your Diet . . . one-third of this quota in each category.

FATS should preferably be cold-pressed (not hydrogenated) vegetable oils, which are unsaturated fats . . . although a minimum of animal fat (saturated) such as unsalted butter may be used.

STARCHES are primarily whole grain breads and cereals and potatoes.

Pure, natural honey is the finest source of NATURAL SUGAR. Dates, which have a high concentration of natural sugar also count in this category . . . so when you include dates in your fresh fruits, cut down on the honey.

RE-EDUCATE YOUR TASTE BUDS

You will be amazed at how many different and delicious menus you can work out by following this basic Program of Natural Nutrition. You are in for a taste-treat adventure as well as a wonderful adventure in health . . . and as a guide, let me refer you to our *Bragg Complete Health Gourmet Recipe Book, which contains more than 1,000 flavorful, healthful recipes garnered from many parts of world, and our Vegetarian No-Salt, No-Sugar Recipe Book,* which contains nutritious, delicious recipes! (See back pages for ordering information.)

At first it may take some willpower to make the transition from dead to live foods, because your taste has been distorted by salt and other condiments. But as your 260 taste buds recover from salt paralysis and come alive again, you will find new and unexpected delights in relishing the true, natural flavors of the foods you eat. Powdered kelp makes an excellent salt substitute without paralyzing the taste buds. You can acquire skill in the use of healthful herbs which enhance natural flavors, as the great French chefs do.

Best of all, not only will you enjoy your food more . . . you will also find a greater joy in living. There is no substitute for the glorious feeling of vitality and energy that comes from a healthy body!

THE LAW OF SUPPLY AND DEMAND

It is well worth the time and effort to read food labels, discard the dead foods, and insist on fresh, live foods from reliable sources. I travel around the world on my lecture tours, and over the years I have always been able to find enough fresh, natural foods to maintain my Live Food Diet, wherever I may be. If you know what to look for, you can find it.

What the consumer demands, long enough and loudly enough, the market supplies. Today . . . probably because so many people feel sick or half-sick . . . there is a growing awareness of the importance of healthful nutrition . . . and an increasing supply of natural foods in general markets as well as in Health Food Stores.

In an implicit repudiation of his own products, billionaire food processor H. L. Hunt made front page news (LOS ANGELES TIMES, Sept. 16, 1972) with his own personal health food diet! A large photograph showed the 83-year-old Texas oil and commercial food magnate, reputed to be one of the richest men in the world, crawling around on all fours (knees bent) demonstrating the creeping exercise he takes daily to strengthen his back muscles after injury in an automobile accident.

Then, according to the Associated Press report, this man who has made a great part of his fortune from the processed and canned foods which bear his name . . . and labels listing the ingredients, including preservatives . . . demonstrated and expounded upon his own personal diet of fresh fruit and juices, nuts and fresh vegetables, grown in his own garden. He stated that these should be eaten raw, without salt . . . and that he avoids white flour and white sugar, eating cracked wheat homemade bread and honey.

Is it too much to hope for that someday a giant food processor such as this will extend his concern for his own personal health to concern for the health of the consumers of his products?

The same inventive technology . . . which created the new problems of malnutrition in solving the old problems of transportation and storage . . . has within itself the power to solve both the old and the new problems of nutrition in a healthful way. The development of refrigeration methods and increasingly rapid transport now make it possible and feasible for fresh foods to be brought to the marketplaces of the world in their natural state, without destroying the natural vitamins, minerals and other vital nutrients.

This, of course, would mean that large food refining and processing plants would become obsolete . . . and therefore food manufacturers would undergo an interim loss while converting to methods that would benefit the health of the consumer. This will not be done until the demand for healthful, natural foods becomes so great that major suppliers will have to fill it, or risk a permanent instead of a temporary loss.

The law of supply and demand is a natural law ... and it always works, sooner or later. Already the trend is showing. As you and others join the ranks of those of us who demand natural, live foods, the supply will increase. And so will the health of our country and our civilization.

OSTEOPOROSIS DUE TO FAULTY DIET

Remember that the bones which comprise your spinal column and the rest of your skeletal system are living tissue ... and must receive the proper nourishment in order to be strong and healthy.

Basic bone structure, as we discussed previously, consists of a rigid outer sheath which gives the bone its shape and strength, filled with elastic, spongy material called marrow. Engineers have adapted this structural principle in the construction of buildings, finding that such supports as metal pipes filled with dirt, for example, are stronger, more enduring and resilient than solid, rigid structures. These man-made structures, however, deteriorate with time. Not so, the living bones of the human skeleton.

Our bones do not "grow brittle with age" ... they become brittle, weak and porous because of deficiences in diet. This condition is known as osteoporosis (osteo = bone; porosis = full of holes, or porous).

Although osteoporosis has long been considered an almost inevitable affliction of people over 50 years of age, the time element is not the basic factor. It is true that the longer you abuse your body by incorrect diet, inadequate exercise and insufficient rest, the greater the price you will pay in the degenerative symptoms commonly known as "aging." But this can happen at any stage of your calendar years. Look at the number of young men and women who are rejected from the armed services and from civilian work requiring good physical stamina, because of various physical deficiences from "fallen arches" to curvature of the spine ... due, in my opinion, primarily to the habitual American "trash" diet of commercialized "dead" foods.

When I was doing nutritional research along the Adriatic coast of Italy, I found "ageless" men and women who were well advanced in calendar years but whose bodies were supple and whose bones were firm, strong and resilient. Their diet consisted primarily of organically grown, properly cooked vegetables and natural cheeses ... rich in natural vitamins and minerals ... the cheeses also being a prime source of protein and calcium, essential for strong bones. In fact, in my extensive research on nutrition, I have never found osteoporosis among any people who lived on a diet of "live" natural foods.

In addition to the lack of essential vitamins and minerals, the general American diet is also highly acid-producing ... due to the high proportion of refined white sugar, refined white flour and animal proteins, which increase the acidity of the human system with an adverse effect on the bones. Strong bones require an alkaline balance in the body metabolism, naturally maintained by a higher proportion of raw fruits and vegetables in the diet.

The worst villain is refined white sugar and its products ... there is no single material that is so devastating to the spine and other bones of the body. It leaches the calcium, phosphorus, magnesium and manganese out of the bones ... making them weak, porous and brittle. Candy and sweets and other refined white sugar products are well known as prime causes of tooth decay. Since teeth are the hardest tissue in the human body, you can well understand what refined white sugar does to the other bones and cartilages of the rest of the skeletal system, including your vital spinal column.

YOUR SPINE NEEDS THESE ORGANIC MINERALS

The only way to protect yourself against osteoporosis ... or to restore weak, porous, brittle bones to a healthy state ... is by proper nutrition. Given the proper tools to work with, the human body is self-healing and self-repairing. But don't expect overnight miracles. If you have been eating incorrectly for a period of time, it is going to take time to repair the damage after you make the change to a Program of Natural Nutrition. Start today! Eliminate the dead foods from your diet ... and give your bones and the rest of your body the live foods on which they will thrive.

For strong, healthy bones and a spinal column that can really serve its purpose as the mainspring of your body, particular attention should be paid to the foods which supply the organic minerals essential to bone-building. These are Calcium, Phosphorus, Magnesium and Manganese.

POSTURE CHART (Grade Yourself)

GRADE 1 POINT FOR EACH BOX	GOOD	FAIR	POOR
HEAD			
SHOULDERS			
SPINE			
HIPS			
ANKLES			
NECK			
UPPER BACK			
TRUNK			
ABDOMEN			
LOWER BACK			
TOTAL SCORES			

CALCIUM, which is important in the repair of all body cells, is the major component of the bones of the body. Ninety percent of the body's calcium is to be found in the skeletal system, where it is not only utilized as the main ingredient of bone structure but also stored for use elsewhere in the body as needed. If your diet is deficient in natural, organic calcium, your bones will not only suffer from this lack but will become further weakened by the drain on their inadequate supply for other uses throughout the body.

Although only 1% of the body's calcium is used by the soft tissues, it is vital to health, especially of the nerves. Not only your spinal column but also your spinal cord needs this organic mineral. The most noticeable sign of calcium deficiency is extreme nervousness. Without the proper amount of calcium in the blood, the nerves cannot send messages. Tension and strain result. It is impossible for the body to relax. This is apparent in children who are highly emotional. It shows first in a mean and unpleasant disposition, fretful crying and temper tantrums, later developing into muscular twitching, spasms and even convulsions.

Both adults and children reveal calcium deficiencies by nervous habits such as biting the fingernails and restless movements of hands and feet, irritability and "jumpiness." Calcium deficiency can be a major contributing cause of adverse personality changes.

Fortunately, an adequate supply of calcium in the system has the opposite effect. In my long experience as a nutritionist, I have seen the meanest, grouchiest, most irritable, nervous people make a personality change upward . . . a transformation into happy, friendly, self-reliant people . . . by following the natural laws of proper nutrition and healthful living.

Natural Sources of Calcium offer such a wide variety that this important mineral can be included in a different way at every meal. Protein foods rich in Calcium include organ meats such as liver, kidneys, heart, etc.; natural, unprocessed yellow cheeses; fresh, fertile eggs. Stone ground cornmeal, whole natural oatmeal and whole natural barley are fine sources. So are raw nuts and seeds. Green leafy vegetables abound in Calcium . . . alfalfa sprouts, artichokes, beet greens, mustard greens, kale, cabbage, cauliflower, dandelion greens, green lettuce . . . as well as carrots and cucumbers. Fruit sources include oranges, sun-dried dates, figs and raisins.

PHOSPHORUS combines with Calcium and Vitamins A and D in proper proportion for balanced bone structure and body metabolism.

Natural Sources include tongue, sweetbreads, all organ meats . . . fish and codliver oil . . . natural cheese . . . soybeans, raw spinach, cucumbers, alfalfa sprouts, peas, kale, mustard greens, watercress . . . brazil nuts . . . whole grain rye, whole wheat, bran . . . raw wheat germ.

MAGNESIUM is necessary for Calcium and Vitamin D metabolism in helping to build and prevent the softening of bones.

Natural Sources are string beans, peas, garbanzos, kidney beans, dried lima beans . . . brussels sprouts, chard, cucumbers, alfalfa sprouts, raw spinach . . . bran and whole wheat . . . avocados . . . pine nuts and sunflower seeds . . . prunes and raisins . . . honey.

MANGANESE is an important trace mineral which serves as a carrier of oxygen from the blood to the cells. It is particularly important in the nourishment of the intervertebral disks and cartilage which have no direct blood circulation.

Natural Sources include liver, fertile egg yolk, fish, poultry, organ meats, all natural cheeses . . . agar, dulse, kelp . . . potatoes, especially the skins (boil or bake in jackets and eat skin) . . . lettuce, watercress, celery, onions . . . alfalfa sprouts, peas, beans of all kinds . . . bran and natural cornmeal . . . almonds, filberts, chestnuts, walnuts . . . bananas.

Remember that your body must have organic minerals . . . i.e., from plant or animal sources. No member of the animal kingdom can assimilate inorganic minerals as they come directly from the earth. Only plants can digest inorganic minerals, and transform these into organic form which can be utilized by animals and humans.

So, if you take mineral supplements, make sure these are from organic sources. To take inorganic calcium tablets, for example, would not supply your bones with the calcium they need . . . it would only clog up your system with indigestible chalk. Bone meal is the finest supplementary source of calcium and other organic minerals essential for strong, healthy bones.

VITAMINS ESSENTIAL TO A HEALTHY SPINE

All the natural vitamins are important for health. Of special importance to a healthy spine are Vitamins A, C and D for building and maintaining strong, resilient bone structure. The B-Complex Vitamins are essential to the spinal cord and nervous system.

VITAMINS A and D are essential in regulating the use of calcium and phosphorus in the body, the two major elements in the formation, building and maintenance of the bones . . . and vital to the efficient functioning of the nervous system. Vitamins A and D act together as catalysts in this all-important phase of body metabolism. Without them, the parathyroid glands of the endocrine system cannot carry out their primary function of maintaining the balanced interaction and distribution of calcium and phosphorus . . . and both bones and nerves deteriorate. There is a marked drop in bone density in people whose diet has been deficient in Vitamins A and D over a period of time. Abnormal spaces appear in the bone structure, and the bone cells become thin, brittle and chalky . . . osteoporosis.

Natural Sources of Vitamin A are colored fruits and vegetables such as carrots, yams, yellow squash, papaya, apricots, peaches, melons . . . dairy products . . . fertile fresh eggs . . . liver . . . fish liver oils.

Natural Sources of Vitamin D also include fish liver oils, unsaturated fats, fertile fresh eggs, whole milk and butter . . . but the prime source is sunshine. A daily sunbath will supply your quota of Vitamin D, and improve your health in many other ways as well. Give your body time to absorb Vitamin D through the skin before washing off perspiration after a sunbath.

VITAMIN C supplies collagen, which is the adhesive substance that holds together all the cells in all the bones and nerves and other tissues of the body. Without Vitamin C, we would literally "fall apart." Since this vital vitamin is not stored by the body, we need a constant supply of Vitamin C in the daily diet.

Natural Sources are citrus fruits, berries, greens, cabbage, sweet green bell peppers. These should be eaten raw and fresh, as Vitamin C is easily destroyed by cooking.

B-COMPLEX VITAMINS include:

Vitamin B-1 . . . Thiamine, or thiamine chloride, often called the "anti-neuritic" or "anti-berberi" vitamin, aids growth and digestion and is essential for normal functioning of nerve tissues, muscles and heart. Signs of deficiency include nervous irritability, insominia, loss of weight and appetite, weakness and lassitude, mental depression.

Vitamin B-2 . . . Riboflavin, or Vitamin G, promotes general health and particularly affects health of the eyes, mouth and skin. Deficiency is often evidenced in itching, burning or bloodshot eyes, inflammation of the mouth, purplish tongue, cracking of corners of the lips.

Vitamin B-6 . . . Pyridoxine, prevents various nervous and skin disorders, aids in food assimilation and in protein and fat metabolism. Nervousness, insomnia, skin eruption and loss of muscular control are signs of deficiency.

Vitamin B-12 . . . Cobalomin, commonly known as "the great red vitamin," aids in the formation and regeneration of red blood cells (manufactured in the bone marrow) and is thus essential in prevention of anemia. It also promotes growth and increased appetite in children, and acts as a general tonic for adults. Deficiency may lead to nutritional and pernicious anemias, with fatigue as a major symptom. Growth failure and poor appetite are among deficiency signs in children.

Natural Sources of B-Complex Vitamins . . . It is important to include the entire B-Complex in your diet, and Nature has provided for this. Brewer's yeast heads the list of B-rich foods, closely followed by raw wheat germ and beef liver, both fresh and desiccated. Other organ meats, especially beef heart and brains and lamb kidney, are good sources . . . as well as lean beef and pork . . . fresh, fertile eggs, especially the yolk . . . fish . . . natural cheeses. Natural, unsalted peanut butter (not hydrogenated) is an excellent source of B-Complex Vitamins . . . so are raw and fresh roasted peanuts. Whole grains such as barley, and 100% whole grain flours such as buckwheat flour, cornmeal, etc., are included . . . as well as oatmeal and rice husks. Vegetable sources include raw and dried beans such as lima and soya beans, green beans . . . raw and dried green peas . . . and leafy green vegetables such as collards, turnip greens, mustard greens, spinach, broccoli, cabbage. B-rich fruits are oranges, grapefruit, bananas, avocados, cantaloupe. Natural molasses is a fine source. Alone or with other dishes, mushrooms add flavor and B Vitamins. Chicken and such shellfish as lobster, oysters and crab meat are on the B-Complex list.

If you are suffering from a deficiency of these vitamins . . . and most Americans are . . . it might be wise to add natural vitamin supplements until you overcome the deficiencies. Be sure that these vitamin supplements are from organic natural sources, as the synthetic vitamins are not so well assimilated by the body . . . nor can we be sure that the synthetic substitutes contain the same vital elements as the natural vitamins.

A NOTE ABOUT MILK

Milk . . . both cow's milk and goat's milk . . . and milk products are excellent sources of protein, calcium, phosphorus, A, D and B-Complex vitamins. This includes certified raw milk, fresh whole or skim milk, buttermilk, and skim powdered milk, as well as cottage cheese, yoghurt and natural yellow cheeses.

In the foregoing lists of Natural Sources, I have stressed cheeses rather than milk itself because cheeses are well assimilated into the body metabolism of both children and adults.

Milk is better suited to the growing period of children and youths, and should form an important part of their diet. During growth, the human body is "programmed" to utilize fully the vital nutritive elements as they are contained in milk . . . the proteins, organic minerals, vitamins, natural sugars and other nutrients . . . which are needed for normal development.

After full growth is attained, however, certain chemical changes take place in the body metabolism. Calcium, for example, is needed in greater proportion during the growth period than it is after the skeleton is stabilized in size. For adults, therefore, cheese is preferable to milk as a source of calcium which can be readily assimilated and used in the body . . . while a growing child can assimilate both milk and cheese.

The same principle holds true throughout the animal kingdom. The young are nourished on their mother's milk during the period of rapid growth and body development. Then their diet naturally changes to satisfy the needs of the semi-mature and mature animal. My experience during a lifetime as a nutritionist and bio-chemist leads me to conclude that this principle also applies to humans.

DON'T STIFFEN YOUR JOINTS

Proper nutrition is as important as proper exercise for a strong, supple spine. Even the Spine Motion Exercises cannot achieve permanent effectiveness if you allow the vertebral joints to become stiffened and calcified with inorganic minerals and toxic acid crystals from improper eating and drinking habits.

As noted, the average civilized diet is highly acid in content, upsetting the natural alkaline-acid balance of the body. After each meal, an indigestible toxic residue remains . . . which takes the form of toxic acid crystals, inorganic calcium-like mineral substances that cannot be absorbed by the body. And where do these toxic acid crystals go?

66

Remember, the movable joints of the skeletal system, including those of the spinal column, are lubricated with synovial fluid which, under normal conditions, is ample to last a lifetime. But this space between the joints offers the easiest location for deposit of the indigestible toxic acid crystals. Gradually the synovial fluid is displaced by these calcified substances, and the joints become stiff and painful. A

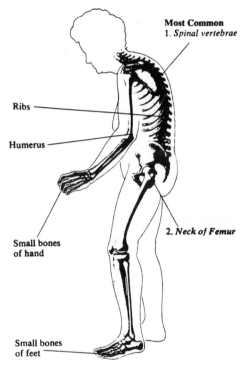

Most Common
1. *Spinal vertebrae*

Ribs

Humerus

Small bones
of hand

2. *Neck of Femur*

Small bones
of feet

LOCATIONS IN THE BODY
WHERE MISERY HITS THE HARDEST.

24 million Americans have osteoporsis which means your bones are porous (holes), more brittle and breakable! This calls for an immediate lifestyle change to 100% health to help eliminate and reverse the problem. How? By improving your diet with more healthy fiber, whole grains, oat bran, fresh fruits, vegetables, sprouts, beans, brown rice, raw seeds, and nuts. Reduce animal proteins for it lowers your calcium levels. Get regular exercise for its revitalizing and promotes healthier bones. Sunshine (vitamin D) in sensible doses is important for healthy bones and makes a big difference to one's health! Not only do you need to get ample minerals from your foods, but take a good, vitamin-mineral supplement daily to insure that you're getting all the necessary nutrients. Researchers state that women over 40 need 1,500 mgs of calcium daily, plus 3 mgs of the trace mineral Boron.

movable joint is the one place in the body where you don't want calcium! . . . especially inorganic calcium, which replaces the lubricating synovial fluid with a kind of cement. The intervertebral disks are also subject to this type of calcification.

This is one of the main reasons why it is so important for you to follow the Basic Rules of Natural Nutrition which I have outlined for you. If you plan your menus along these lines, you will maintain a diet with the proper alkaline-acid balance . . . which is about 3/5 alkaline and 2/5 acid. In general, fruits and vegetables (with a few exceptions) are alkaline forming . . . while proteins, starches, fats and sugars are acid forming.

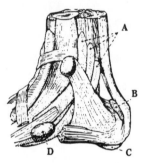

DEPOSITS OF INORGANIC MINERALS AND TOXIC ACID CRYSTALS IN THE HEEL OF THE FOOT CAUSING GREAT PAIN!

A. Inorganic minerals deposited under the tendons.

B. Under the tendon of Achilles.

C. Under the heel.

D. Under the middle foot.

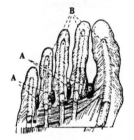

INORGANIC MINERAL DEPOSITS THAT MAY DEPOSIT THEMSELVES BETWEEN THE BONES OF THE TOES (A, B,) CAUSING STIFFNESS IN THE FEET.

Bragg Health Pep Drink

Prepare in blender, add 1 ice cube if desired chilled:

Juice of 2-3 Oranges (fresh) or	*1/2 tsp. Vitamin C Powder*
unsweetened Pineapple Juice	*1/3 tsp. pure Pectin Powder*
or 1 glass Distilled Water	*1-2 Bananas, Ripe*
1 tbsp. Raw Wheat Germ	*1/3 tsp. Flaxseed oil*
1 tsp. Brewers Yeast	*1 tsp. Honey*
1 tbsp. Raw Oat Bran	*1 tbsp. Soy Protein Powder*
1 tbsp. Lecithin Granules	*1 tsp. Raw Sunflower or*
1/2 tsp. Raisins	*Pumpkin Seeds*

Optional:
4 Apricots (sun dried, unsulphered). Soak in jar overnight in distilled water or unsweetened pineapple juice. We soak enough to last for several days. Keep refrigerated. NOTE: In summer you can add fresh fruit in season—peaches, strawberries, berries, apricots or any other fresh fruit in season instead of the banana. In winter try (sugar-free) frozen fruits.

DRINK ONLY DISTILLED WATER

Not only the food you eat . . . but also the very water you drink . . . can add to the accumulation of "cementing" substances in your vertebrae and other movable joints throughout your body.

Remember that the body cannot digest or absorb inorganic minerals. Unfortunately, most of the drinking water of the world contains such minerals, to a greater or lesser degree. Hard water has the heaviest natural concentration of inorganic minerals. The purifying agents used in the water supplies of most towns and cities, although these kill bacteria and germs, add more inorganic substances including harsh chemicals. Nor do "water softeners" help this condition . . . in fact, they aggravate it by adding salt, another harmful inorganic mineral.

Naturally soft water such as rain or snow water is ideal drinking water in its pure state, but today that occurs only in isolated areas. The air over populated areas of the world, especially where there is industry and motorized transportation, is now so contaminated that rain and snow become polluted as they pass through the air from clouds to earth.

The only safe drinking water today is distilled water, preferably steam distilled. Pure, fresh fruit and vegetable juices also fall in this category, as these contain Nature's own distilled water.

For a thorough analysis and discussion of this vital subject, read our book on *THE SHOCKING TRUTH ABOUT WATER* (See back pages for ordering)

In the Bragg household . . . as well as on our world-wide lecture tours . . . we use only steam distilled water for drinking and cooking. For a strong, flexible spine . . . supple joints . . . and general good health . . . I heartily recommend that you do likewise. Bottles of distilled water are available in most markets . . . or you can arrange to have it delivered to your home, and even have a water cooler installed to make it easier for you and your family to drink pure water.

The best method, of course, is to install a simple, easy-to-use Steam Water Distiller in your home. Information on reliable processes and equipment may be obtained without charge from: Pure Water Systems Research, 7340 Hollister Ave. Goleta, California 93117

The hardest thing of all in life—The conquest not of time and space, but of ourselves, of our stupidity and inertia, of our greediness and touchiness, of our fear and intolerant dogmatism.

FASTING CLEANSES THE BODY

Once every week I take a 24-hour distilled water fast . . . giving my digestive, circulatory and eliminative systems a rest from the usual assimilation and distribution of food . . . and releasing that vital energy to be used in a thorough housecleaning, ridding my body of all toxic poisons. Yes, even living the strictly natural health life that I do, I find this weekly fast highly beneficial. Several times a year I take a longer fast of seven days.

Fasting is Nature's way of helping the body to keep itself in good repair and to heal itself. Animals instinctively refuse to eat when they are sick or disturbed.

But the average human has a preconceived notion that if he skips a few meals, dangerous things will happen to his body. Nothing is farther from the truth! I have supervised fasts for thousands of health students, who have made fasting the first major step on the Road to Health, and have seen people benefit from distilled water fasts up to 30 days. I do not, however, advise anyone to take a prolonged fast without professional supervision, which can be obtained at Health Spas in many parts of the world. On your own, you may safely begin with one day per week.

A weekly fast of 24 hours on distilled water only, flavored with a little lemon juice if you wish, will help you greatly in making the transition from incorrect habits of eating and living into a program of proper nutrition and exercise. It will help your body to rid itself of accumulated toxic poisons . . . to flush out the calcified acid crystals from your joints. But don't expect your first fast to cleanse you completely! Although you are probably unaware of it, you have been clogging your body with poisonous residue for whatever period of time you have been eating "dead" foods. It will take time to get these toxins out of your system.

But the reward will be well worth the effort. As you feel new life and vigor surging through your body . . . when you finally experience that glorious state of being known as perfect health . . . you will begin to enjoy living as never before!

At first, during this transition, you are likely to experience certain discomfort . . . symptoms similar to what is called "a bad cold." This is known as a "healing crisis" . . . the natural reaction of your body when its vital energy is released to cleanse itself. As a matter of fact, a "cold" is actually a healing crisis induced by Nature herself, when the accumulation of toxic poisons in the body has reached such a dangerous point that the body's own alarm signals trigger emergency action. The discharges of mucus through the nose, mouth and bowels are the body's natural methods of ridding itself of these poisons. Let Nature take her course, and work with her by resting and fasting on distilled water. If the healing crisis is prolonged, you may add fresh fruit juices and/or herb teas ... but do not add to the burden of your body's housecleaning by stuffing yourself with food. You will feel infinitely better afterward.

To fast intelligently and with real benefit, you should follow the instructions in my book, *THE MIRACLE OF FASTING*. This will explain how to take a fast, how to break a fast, and what physical reactions to expect while fasting.

USE YOUR "BACKBONE" FOR PHYSICAL FITNESS

In carrying out this Program of Physical Fitness with Spine Motion, you must use your "backbone" ... in both senses of the word! In the folklore sense of "courage" and "willpower" you must exercise your "backbone" to transform your pattern of life from one of merely tolerable existence to living in the full joy of radiant health. Particularly in the beginning, you will need mental discipline and willpower to "re-program" your habits of diet, posture and physical exercise in accordance with the Natural Laws of Health, as outlined in this book.

Vital in this transformation is the literal exercise of your "backbone" ... stretching and strengthening your spinal column with the unique Bragg Spine Motion Exercises ... as well as the Posture and Strengthening Exercises ... according to the instructions I have given you.

Do the exercises in this book slowly for the first week or so. Feel your way along so as not to get your muscles sore with too vigorous contractions at first. Always exercise short of the point of pain. But don't stop your daily routine! A slight soreness is natural when your muscles have been unused ... but it will disappear as you continue your program.

Remember, if you can move a muscle you can strengthen it. I have never seen anyone who could move a muscle and was willing to really exercise every day who couldn't develop a limber and supple spine ... gain added strength ... and have a more active life! And look better, feel better, and get more real enjoyment out of living.

Never forget ... if you don't use your spine, you will lose it. It will become prematurely old, stiff and painful. The body and spine remain youthful and strong only with use!

YOU ARE AS OLD AND AS YOUNG AS YOUR SPINE

No matter how you have neglected and abused your spine, by following the instructions given in this book you can reverse the condition. The recuperative powers of the human body are tremendous. The body is self-repairing and self-healing.

But you must give your body the natural aids it needs. It can only repair and restore itself to health when the correct nutrition and exercise are provided.

Let me repeat, the body remains strong only if it is used. More than 70% of the people in physicians' offices today have under-exercised spines. Your body and your spine need daily exercise.

Make your Spinal Exercises a regular part of your daily activities ... just like brushing your teeth and combing your hair every morning.

And don't tell me you "don't have time" to have a limber spine and a physically fit body! That's absolute nonsense. If you have a sense of true values, you will find the time to take care of your precious body. It's the only one you'll ever get.. . . so take extra special care of it! It will reward you with a bright and healthy life.

Within a few weeks of following the program outlined in this book, your spine will feel flexible and supple. You will walk with a spring in your step. You will feel the vital energy surging over your body. You will be surprised just how wonderful you will feel when you get the spine limbered up! You will find that you do not tire so easily. You will have more "go-power" and energetic drive.

And it will not stop there. Each day you will add new zest ... new vigor and power to your body. Remember, the world is alive, and you're alive. And you are never too old to be young! This is a great time to be fully alive with an "ageless" body.

Now get started and really begin to feel fully alive again! You will be mighty happy you read this book. Like thousands of others you will get a new lease on life as you follow this Fitness Program with Spine Motion. Life can really be a joy when the spine is functioning perfectly.

Paul C. Bragg   Patricia Bragg

72

WHEN YOU ARE HEALTHY — YOU ARE HAPPY!

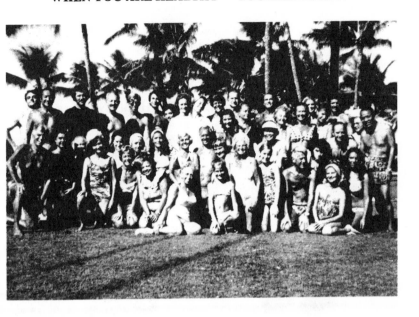

JOIN THE FUN AT THE BRAGG "LONGER LIFE, HEALTH & HAPPINESS CLUB" WHEN YOU VISIT HAWAII – IT'S FREE!

Paul C. Bragg, daughter Patricia and their wonderful healthy members of the Bragg "Longer Life, Health and Happiness Club" exercise daily at the beautiful Fort DeRussy lawn, at the world famous Waikiki Beach in Honolulu, Hawaii.

Membership is free and open to everyone who wishes to attend any morning – Monday through Saturday, from 9:00 to 10:30 a.m. for deep breathing, exercising, meditation, group singing. And on Saturday, after the class – health lectures on how to live a long, healthy life!

The group averages 75 to 125 per day, according to the seasons. From December to March it can go up to 200. When away lecturing, their dedicated leaders carry on until their return. Thousands have visited the club from around the world and then carry the message of health and fitness to friends and relatives back home.

Patricia extends an invitation to you and your friends to join the club for wholesome, healthy fellowship . . . when you visit Honolulu, Hawaii. Be sure also to visit the outer Hawaiian Islands (Maui, Kauai, Hawaii, Molakai) for a fulfilling, healthy vacation.

PURE WATER (H$_2$O) A PRIME REQUISITE OF HEALTH

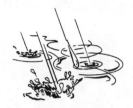

THE 65% WATERY HUMAN

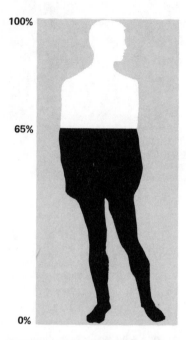

100%

65%

0%

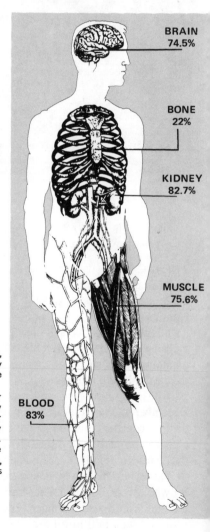

**BRAIN
74.5%**

**BONE
22%**

**KIDNEY
82.7%**

**MUSCLE
75.6%**

**BLOOD
83%**

THE 65% WATERY HUMAN

The amount of water in the human body, averaging 65 per cent, varies considerably from person to person and even from one part of the body to another (right). A lean man may have as much as 70 per cent of his weight in the form of body water, while a woman, because of her larger proportion of water-poor fatty tissues, may be only 52 per cent water. The lowering of the water content in the blood is what triggers the hypothalamus, the brain's thirst center to send out its familiar demand for a drink.

"Water Is The Best Drink For A Wise Man" — Henry Thoreau

PURE WATER — ESSENTIAL FOR HEALTH!

Distilled water is one of the world's best and purest waters! It is excellent for detoxification and fasting programs and for helping clean out all the cells, organs, and fluids of the body because it can help carry away so many harmful substances!

Water from chemically-treated public water systems and even from many wells and springs is likely to be loaded with poisonous chemicals and toxic trace elements.

Depending upon the kind of piping that the water has been run through, the water in our homes, offices, schools, hospitals, etc., is likely to be overloaded with zinc (from old-fashioned galvanized pipes) or with copper and cadmium (from copper pipes). These trace elements are released in excessive quantity by the chemical action of the water on the metals of the water pipes.

Yes, pure water is essential for health, either from the natural juices of vegetables, fruits, and other foods, or from the water of high purity obtained by steam distillation which is the best method, or by one of the new high-efficiency deionization processes.

The body is constantly working for you . . . breaking down old bone and tissue cells and replacing them with new ones. As the body casts off the old minerals and other products of broken-down cells, it must obtain new supplies of the essential elements for the new cells. Moreover, Scientists are only now beginning to understand that various kinds of dental problems, different types of arthritis, and even some forms of hardening of the arteries are due to varying kinds of imbalances in the levels of calcium, phosphorus, and magnesium in the body. Disorders can also be caused by imbalances in the ratios of various minerals to each other.

Each individual healthy body requires a proper balance within itself of all the nutritive elements. It is just as bad for any individual to have too much of one item as it is to have too little of that one or of another one. It takes appropriate levels of phosphorus and magnesium to keep calcium in solution so it can be formed into new cells of bone and teeth. Yet, there must not be too much of those nor too little calcium in the diet, or old bone will be taken away but new bone will not be formed.

In addition, we now know that diets which are unbalanced and inappropriate for a given individual can deplete the body of calcium, magnesium, potassium, and other major and minor elements.

Diets which are high in meats, fish, eggs, grains, nuts, seeds, or their products may provide unbalanced excesses of phosphorus which will deplete calcium and magnesium from the bones and tissues of the body and cause them to be lost in the urine.

A diet high in fats will tend to increase the uptake of phosphorus from the intestines relative to calcium and other basic minerals. Such a high-fat diet can produce losses of calcium, magnesium, and other basic minerals in the same way a high-phosphorus diet does.

Diets excessively high in fruits or their juices may provide unbalanced excesses of potassium in the body, and calcium and magnesium will again be lost from the body through the urine.

Deficiencies of calcium and magnesium . . . for example can produce all kinds of problems in the body ranging from dental decay and osteoporosis to muscular cramping, hyper-activity, muscular twitching, poor sleep patterns, and excessive frequency of uncontrolled patterns of urination. Similarly, deficiencies of other minerals, or imbalances in the levels of those minerals, can produce many other problems in the body.

Therefore, it is important to clean and detoxify the body through fasting and through using distilled or other pure water as well as healthy organically-grown vegetable and fruit juices. At the same time, it is also important to provide the body with adequate sources of new minerals. This can be done by eating a widely-distributed diet of wholesome vegetables, including kelp and other sea vegetables for adults and healthy mother's milk for infants, and certified raw goat's or cow's milk for those children and adults who are not adversely affected by milk products . . . but most processed home homogenized milks we do not suggest using.

But, despite dietary sources such as these, many adults and children in so-called civilized cultures will be found to have low levels of essential minerals in their bodies due to losses caused by coffee, tea, carbonated beverages, and long-term bad diets containing too much sugar and other sweets as well as products made from refined flours and containing refined table salt.

In addition, the body's organ systems can be thrown out of balance by continuing stress, by toxins in our air and water, by disease-produced injuries, and by pre-natal deficiencies in the mother's diet or life style.

As a result, many, if not most people in our so-called civilization may need to take mineral supplements such as the new chelated multiple mineral preparations as well as a broad-range multiple-vitamin tablet.

BORON – MIRACLE TRACE MINERAL FOR HEALTHY BONES

BORON – Trace mineral for healthy bones helps the body have more Calcium, Mineral & Hormones! Boron is found in vegetables, fruits, nut and especially good sources are broccoli, prunes, dates, raisins, almonds, peanuts and soybeans.

Take time
for **12** things

1 Take time to Work—
   it is the price of success.

2 Take time to Think—
   it is the source of power.

3 Take time to Play—
   it is the secret of youth.

4 Take time to Read—
   it is the foundation of knowledge.

5 Take time to Worship—
   it is the highway of reverance and washes the
   dust of earth from our eyes.

6 Take time to Help and Enjoy Friends—
   it is the source of happiness.

7 Take time to Love—
   it is the one sacrament of life.

8 Take time to Dream—
   it hitches the soul to the stars.

9 Take time to Laugh—
   it is the singing that helps with life's loads.

10 Take time for Beauty—
   it is everywhere in nature.

11 Take time for Health—
   it is the true wealth and treasure of life.

12 Take time to Plan—
   it is the secret of being able to have time to
   take time for the first eleven things.

Every man is the builder of a temple called his body . . . We are all sculptors and painters, and our material is our own flesh and blood and bones. Any nobleness begins at once to refine a man's features, any meanness or sensuality to imbrute them.
                                                    - Henry David Thoreau

IRON-PUMPING OLDSTERS (86 to 96) TRIPLE
THEIR MUSCLE STRENGTH IN 1990 US GOV STUDY

WASHINGTON, June 13, 1990 – Aging nursing home residents, in Boston study, "pumping iron"?

Elderly weight-lifters tripling and quadrupling their muscle strength? Is it possible? Most people would doubt? and wonder?

Government experts on aging gave those questions a resounding "yes" with the results of a new study.

They turned a group of frail Boston nursing-home residents, aged 86 to 96, into weight-lifters to demonstrate that it is never too late to reverse age-related declines in muscle strength. The group participated in a regimen of high-intensity weight-training in a study conducted by the Agriculture Department's Human Nutrition Research Center on Aging at Tufts Unversity in Boston. "A high-intensity weight training program is capable of inducing dramatic increases in muscle strength in frail men and women up to 96 years of age," reported Dr. Maria A. Fiatarone, who headed the study.

AMAZING RESULTS IN 8 WEEKS

"The favorable response to strength training in our subjects was remarkable in light of their very advanced age, extremely sedentary habits, multiple chronic diseases and functional disabilities and nutritional inadequacies.

The elderly weight-lifters increased their muscle strength by anywhere from three-fold to four-fold in as little as eight weeks. Fiatarone said they probably were stronger at the end of the program than they had been in years!

Fiatarone and her associates emphasized the safety of such a closely supervised weight-lifting program, even among people in frail health. The average age of the 10 participants, for instance, was 90. Six had coronary heart disease; seven had arthritis; six had bone fractures resulting from osteoporosis; four had high blood pressure; & all had been physcially inactive for years. Yet no serious medical problems resulted from the program.

A few of the participants did report minor muscle and joint aches, but nine of the 10 completed the program. One man, aged 86, felt a pulling sensation at the site of a previous hernia incision and dropped out after four weeks.

The study participants, drawn from a 712-bed long-term care facility in Boston, worked out three times a week. They performed three sets of eight repetitions with each leg on a weight-lifting machine. The weights were gradually increased from about 10 pounds initially to about 40 pounds at the end of the eight-week program.

Fiatarone said the study carries potentially important implications for older people, who represent a growing proportion of the population. A decline in muscle strength and size is one of the more predictable features of aging.

78

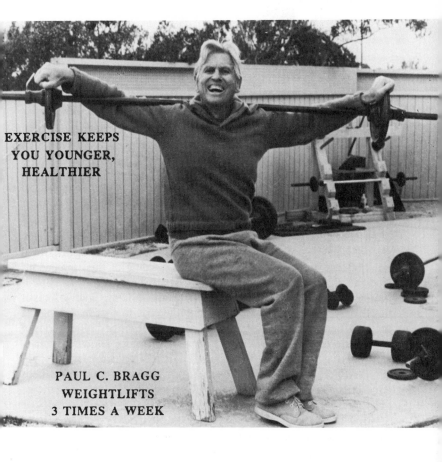

EXERCISE KEEPS
YOU YOUNGER,
HEALTHIER

PAUL C. BRAGG
WEIGHTLIFTS
3 TIMES A WEEK

Muscle strength in the average adult decreases by 30 percent to 50 percent during the course of life. Experts on aging do not know whether the decrease is an unavoidable consequence of aging or results mainly from sedentary lifestyle and other controlable factors.

Muscle atrophy and weakness is not merely a cosmetic problem in elderly people, especially the frail elderly. Researchers have linked muscle weakness with recurrent falls, a major cause of immobility and death in the American elderly population. This is causing millions of dollars yearly in staggering medical costs.

Previous studies have suggested that weight training can be helpful in reversing age-related muscle weakness. But Fiatarone said physicians have been reluctant to recommend weight-lifting for frail elderly with multiple health problems. This new government study might be changing their minds. Also, this study shows the great importance of keeping the 640 body muscles as active and fit as possible to maintain general good health.

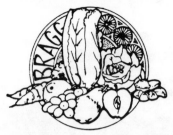

FROM THE AUTHORS

This book was written for YOU. It can be your passport to the Good Life. We Professional Nutritionists join hands in one common objective - high standard of health for all and many added years to your life. Scientific Nutrition points the way - Nature's Way - the only lasting way to build a body free of degenerative diseases and premature aging. This book teaches you how to work with Nature and not against her. Doctors, dentists and others who care for the sick try to repair depleted tissues, which too often mend poorly - if at all. Many of them praise the spreading of this new scientific message of natural foods and methods for long-lasting health and youthfulness at any age. To speed the spreading of this tremendous message, this book was written.

Statements in this book are recitals of scientific findings, known facts of physiology, biological therapeutics and reference to ancient writings as they are found. Paul C. Bragg has been practicing the natural methods of living for over 80 years with highly beneficial results, knowing they are safe and of great value. His daughter Patricia Bragg works with him to carry on the Health Crusade. They make no claims as to what the methods cited in this book will do to one in any given situation, and assume no obligation because of opinions expressed.

No cure for disease is offered in this book. No foods or diets are offered for the treatment or cure of any specific ailment. Nor is it intended as, or to be used as, literature for any food product. Paul C. Bragg and Patricia Bragg express their opinions solely as Public Health Educators, Professional Nutritionists and Teachers.

Certain persons considered experts may disagree with one or more statements in this book, as the same relate to various nutritional recommendations. However, any such statements are considered, nevertheless, to be factual, as based upon long-time experience of Paul C. Bragg and Patricia Bragg in the field of human health.

BRAGG BLESSINGS FROM OUR HOME

From the Bragg home to your home we share our years of health knowledge-years of living close to God and Nature and what joys of fruitful, radiant living this produces-this my Father and I share with you and your loved ones. With Blessing for Health and Happiness,

Patricia Bragg

*Dear friend, I wish above all things that thou may prosper
and be in health even as the soul prospers* - 3 John 2

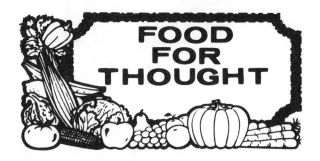

FOOD FOR THOUGHT

Fruit bears the closest relation to light. The sun pours a continuous flood of light into the fruits, and they furnish the best portion of food a human being requires for the sustenance of mind and body. — Alcott

The purest food is fruit, next the cereals, then the vegetables. All pure poets have abstained almost entirely from animal food. Especially should a minister take less meat when he has to write a sermon. The less meat the better sermon. — A. Bronson Alcott

There is much false economy: those who are too poor to have seasonable fruits and vegetables, will yet have pie and pickles all the year. They cannot afford oranges, yet can afford tea and coffee daily. — Health Calendar

The men who kept alive the flame of learning and piety in the Middle Ages were mainly vegetarians. — Sir William Axon

Hearty foods are those in which there is an abundance of potential energy.

If families could be induced to substitute the apple — sound, ripe, and luscious — for the white sugar, whiteflour pies, cakes, candies, and other sweets with which children are too often stuffed, there would be a diminution of doctors' bills, sufficient in a single year to lay up a stock of this delicious fruit for a season's use.

To maintain good health the body must be exercised properly [walking, jogging, deep breathing, good posture, etc.], and nourished wisely [natural foods], so as to provide and increase the good life of joy and happiness. — Paul C. Bragg

Statistics show degenerative ills increasing at alarming rates and attacking people at increasingly early ages. It is time the fact be recognized that diet is largely responsible for this increase, and that sugar, coffee, salt, refined and chemicalized foods, and the lack of exercise are the major culprits.

The lightest breakfast is the best. — Oswald

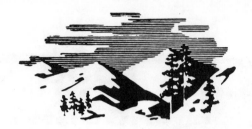

TEN HEALTH COMMANDMENTS

Thou shall respect the body as the highest manifestation of life.

Thou shall abstain from all unnatural, devitalized food and stimulating beverages.

Thou shall nourish thy body with only Natural unprocessed, "live" food, - that . . .

Thou shall extend the years in health for loving, charitable service.

Thou shall regenerate thy body by the right balance of activity and rest.

Thou shall purify thy cells, tissue and blood with pure fresh air and sunshine.

Thou shall abstain from ALL food when out of sorts in mind or body.

Thou shall keep thy thoughts, words and emotions, pure, calm and uplifting.

Thou shall increase thy knowledge of Nature's laws, abide therewith, and enjoy the fruits of thy life's labor.

Thou shall lift up thyself and thy brother man with thine own obedience to God's Natural, Pure Laws of Living.

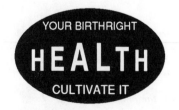

YOUR BIRTHRIGHT
HEALTH
CULTIVATE IT

*"Teach me Thy way, O Lord;
and Lead me in a plain path . . . "*
Psalms 97:11

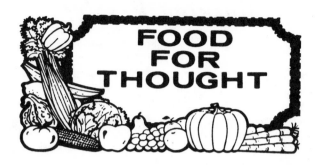

FOOD FOR THOUGHT

Soup rejoices the stomach, and disposes it to receive and digest other food.
— Brillat Savarin

To work the head, temperance must be carried into the diet. — Beecher

To fare well implies the partaking of such food as does not disagree with body or mind. Hence only those fare well who live temperately. — Socrates

The eating of much flesh fills us with a multitude of evil diseases and multitudes of evil desires. — Porphyrises, 233 A.D.

Health is not quoted in the markets because it is without price.

It is a mistake to think that the more a man eats, the fatter and stronger he will become.

The health journals and the doctors all agree that the best and most wholesome part of the New England country doughnut is the hole. The larger the hole, they say, the better the doughnut.

According to the ancient Hindu Scriptures, the proper amount of food is half of what can be conveniently eaten.

The nervousness and peevishness of our times are chiefly attributable to tea and coffee. The digestive organs of confirmed coffee drinkers are in a state of chronic derangement which reacts on the brain, producing fretful and lachrymose moods. — Dr. Bock, 1910

A physician recommended a lady to abandon the use of tea and coffee. "O, but I shall miss it so," said she. "Very likely," replied her medical adviser, "but you are missing health now, and will lose it altogether if you do not."

WATER

To the days of the aged it addeth length;
To the might of the strong it addeth strength;
It freshens the heart, it brightens the sight;
'Tis like quaffing a goblet of morning light.

Morning Resolve

I will this day live a simple, sincere and serene life, repelling promptly every thought of impurity, discontent, anxiety, discouragement and self-seeking. I will cultivate cheerfulness, happiness, charity and the love of brotherhood; exercising economy in expenditure, generosity in giving, carefulness in conversation and diligence in appointed service. I pledge fidelity to every trust and a childlike faith in God, in particular, I will be faithful in those habits of prayer, study, work, physical exercise, deep breathing and good posture. I shall fast one 24 hour period each week, eat only natural foods and get sufficient sleep each night. I will make every effort to improve myself physically, mentally and spiritually every day.

Morning prayer used by Paul C. Bragg and Patricia Bragg

WE THANK THEE

For flowers that bloom about our feet;
    For song of bird and hum of bee;
For all things fair we hear or see,
    Father in heaven we thank Thee!
For blue of stream and blue of sky;
    For pleasant shade of branches high;
For fragrant air and cooling breeze;
    For beauty of the blooming trees,
Father in heaven, we thank Thee!
    For mother-love and father-care,
For brothers strong and sisters fair;
    For love at home and here each day;
For guidance lest we go astray,
    Father in heaven, we thank Thee!
For this new morning with its light;
    For rest and shelter of the night;
For health and food, for love and friends;
    For every thing His goodness sends,
Father in heaven, we thank Thee!

- Ralph Waldo Emerson

PATRICIA BRAGG N.D., Ph.D.
Angel of Health & Healing
Lecturer, Author, Nutritionist, Health Educator & Fitness Advisor to World Leaders, Glamorous Hollywood Stars, Singers, Dancers & Athletes.

Daughter of the world renowned health authority, Paul C. Bragg, Patricia Bragg has on international fame on her own in this field. She conducts Health and Fitness minars for Women's, Men's, Youth and Church Groups throughout the world... and omotes Bragg "How-To, Self-Health" Books in Lectures, on Radio and Television lk Shows throughout the English-speaking world. Consultants to Presidents and oyalty, to the Stars of Stage, Screen and TV and to Champion Athletes, Patricia Bragg d her father are Co-Authors of the Bragg Health Library of Instructive, Inspiring ooks that promote a healthy lifestyle for a long, vital, active life!

Patricia herself is the symbol of perpetual youth and super energy. She is a living d sparkling example of her and her father's healthy lifestyle precepts and this she ares world-wide.

A fifth generation Californian on her mother's side, Patricia was reared by the atural Health Method from infancy. In school, she not only excelled in athletics but so won high honors in her studies and her counseling. She is an accomplished musician d dancer... as well as tennis player, swimmer and mountain climber... and the youngest oman ever to be granted a U.S. Patent. Patricia is a popular gifted Health Teacher and dynamic, in-demand Talk Show Guest where she spreads simple, easy-to-follow alth teachings for everyone.

Man's body is the Temple of the Holy Spirit, and our creator wants us filled with y and Health for a long walk with Him for Eternity. The Bragg Crusade of Health and tness (3 John 2) has carried her around the world... spreading physical, spiritual, notional and mental health and joy. Health is our birthright and Patricia teaches how prevent the destruction of our health from man-made wrong habits of living.

Patricia's been Health Consultant to American Presidents and to the British Royal mily, to Betty Cuthbert, Australia's "Golden Girl" who holds 16 world records and ur Olympic gold medals in women's track and to New Zealand's Olympic Track Star llison Roe. Among those who come to her for advice are some of Hollywood's top stars om Clint Eastwood to the ever youthful singing group The Beach Boys and their milies, singing stars of the Metropolitan Opera and top ballet stars. Patricia's message of world-wide appeal to the people of all ages, nationalities and walks-of-life. Those ho follow the Bragg Health Books & attend the Bragg Crusades are living testimonials ke Super Athlete, Ageless - Jack LaLanne—at age 14 he went from sickness to health.

tricia Bragg inspires you to Renew, Rejuvenate & Revitalize your life with the "Bragg ealthy Lifestyle" Seminars and Lectures world-wide. These are life-changing and illions have benefited with a longer, healthier life! She would love to share her rusade with your organizations, businesses, churches, etc. Also, she is a perfect radio d T.V. talk show guest to spread the message of health and fitness in your area.

Write or call for requests and information:
HEALTH SCIENCE, BOX 7, SANTA BARBARA, CA 93102 1-805-968-1028

PAUL C. BRAGG N.D., Ph.D.

Life Extension Specialist • World Health Crusader
Lecturer and Advisor to Olympic Athletes, Royalty, and Stars

Originator of Health Food Stores - Now World-wide

For almost a Century, Living Proof that his
"Health and Fitness Way of Life" Works Wonders!

Paul C. Bragg is the Father of the Health Movement in America. This dynamic Crusader for worldwide health and fitness is responsible for more "firsts" in the history of Health than any other individual. Here are a few of his incredible pioneering achievements that the world now enjoys:

- Bragg originated, named and opened the first "Health Food Store" in America
- Bragg Crusades pioneered the first Health Lectures across America, inspiring followers to open health stores in cities across the land and now world-wide.
- Bragg introduced pineapple juice and tomato juice to the American public.
- He was the first to introduce and distribute honey nationwide.
- He introduced Juice Therapy in America by importing the first hand-juicers.
- Bragg pioneered Radio Health Programs from Hollywood three times daily.
  Paul and Patricia pioneered a Health TV show from Hollywood to spread "Health and Happiness"... the name of the show! It included exercises, health recipes, visual demonstrations, and guest appearances of famous, health minded people.
- He created the first health foods & products and made them available nation wide: herb teas, health beverages, seven-grain cereals and crackers, health cosmetics, health candies, vitamins and mineral supplements, wheat germ digestive enzymes from papaya, herbs & kelp seasonings, amino acids from soybeans. He inspired others to follow and now thousands of health items are available worldwide.
- He opened the first health restaurants and health spas in America.

Crippled by TB as a teenager, Bragg developed his own eating, breathing and exercising program to rebuild his body into an ageless, tireless, painfree citadel of glowing, radiant health. He excelled in running, swimming, biking, progressive weight training, and mountain-climbing. He made an early pledge to God, in return for his renewed health, to spend the rest of his life showing others the road to health... Paul Bragg made good his pledge!

A living legend and beloved counselor to millions, Bragg was the inspiration and personal advisor on diet and fitness to top Olympic Stars from 4-time swimming Gold Medalist Murray Rose to 3-time track Gold Medalist Betty Cuthbert of Australia, his relative Don Bragg (pole-vaulting Gold Medalist), and countless others. Jack LaLanne, "the original TV King of Fitness," says, "Bragg saved my life at age 14 when I attended the Bragg Crusade in Oakland, California." From the earliest days, Bragg was advisor to the greatest Hollywood Stars, and to giants of American Business. J. C. Penney, Del E. Webb, and Conrad Hilton are just a few that he inspired to long, successful, healthy, active lives!

Dr. Bragg changed the lives of millions worldwide in all walks of life... through his Health Crusades, Books, Tapes and Radio, TV and personal appearances.

HEALTH SCIENCE Box 7, Santa Barbara, California 93102 U.S.A.

SEND FOR IMPORTANT
FREE
HEALTH BULLETINS

Let Patricia Bragg send you, your relatives and friends the latest News Bulletins on Health and Nutrition Discoveries. These are sent periodically. Please enclose two stamps for each U.S.A. name listed. Foreign listings send international postal reply coupons. Please print or type addresses, thank you.

HEALTH SCIENCE Box 7, Santa Barbara, California 93102 U.S.A.

●
_____
Name

_____ (___) _____
Address   Phone

_____
City   State   Zip Code

●
_____
Name

_____ (___) _____
Address   Phone

_____
City   State   Zip Code

●
_____
Name

_____ (___) _____
Address   Phone

_____
City   State   Zip Code

●
_____
Name

_____ (___) _____
Address   Phone

_____
City   State   Zip Code

●
_____
Name

_____ (___) _____
Address   Phone

_____
City   State   Zip Code